Killer Clothes

How Seemingly Innocent Clothing Choices Endanger your Health ... and How to Protect Yourself!

Anna Maria Clement, PhD, NMD, LN
Brian R. Clement, PhD, NMD, LN
Co-Directors, The Hippocrates Health Institute

16
EasyRead Large

RHYW

Copyright Page from the Original Book

Cover design: Jim Scattaregia
Interior design: Jim Scattaregia

Hippocrates Publications, an imprint of Book Publishing Company
P.O. Box 99
Summertown, TN 38483
888-260-8458
www.bookpubco.com

ISBN 13: 978-1-57067-263-7

Printed in the United States

17 16 15 14 13 12 11 9 8 7 6 5 4 3 2 1

Library of Congress Cataloging-in-Publication Data

Clement, Anna Maria.
Killer clothes! : how seemingly innocent clothing choices endanger your health-- and how to protect yourself! / Anna Maria Clement, and Brian R. Clement.
p. cm.
Includes bibliographical references and index.
ISBN 978-1-57067-263-7
1. Textile fibers, Synthetic--Health aspects. 2. Environmental toxicology. I. Clement, Brian R., 1951- II. Title.
RA579.C54 2010
615.9'02--dc22
2010051721

Printed on recycled paper

Book Publishing Company is a member of Green Press Initiative. We chose to print this title on paper with 100% post consumer recycled content, processed without chlorine, which saved the following natural resources:

53 trees
1,460 pounds of solid waste
24,050 gallons of water
4,994 pounds of greenhouse gases
17 million BTU of energy

For more information on Green Press Initiative, visit www.greenpressinitiative.org. Environmental impact estimates were made using the Environmental Defense Fund Paper Calculator. For more information visit www.papercalculator.org.

This optimized ReadHowYouWant edition contains the complete, unabridged text of the original publisher's edition. Other aspects of the book may vary from the original edition.

Set in 16 pt. Verdana

TABLE OF CONTENTS

INTRODUCTION

Why the Emperor Wears No Clothes

As a young girl growing up in Sweden, I (Anna Maria) often heard a Scandinavian folk tale about two swindlers pretending to be weavers who convinced an emperor to purchase clothes made from a material of such high quality that they were "invisible to any man who was unfit for his office or unpardonably stupid." Though the emperor realized that he couldn't see his new clothes, he refused to admit this to anyone out of fear he would be considered stupid or unfit to rule. The emperor's attendants and subjects similarly played along and pretended they could see the clothes.

When the emperor wore his new "clothes" in a public procession, it fell to a little child to exclaim, "He has nothing on at all." This innocent observation broke the spell so that everyone in the kingdom could admit to themselves and to each other that the reported clothes were nothing but a delusion.

This parable, "The Emperor's New Suit," by nineteenth century author Hans Christian Andersen, should hold new levels of meaning for us today. Pride, vanity, and stubborn denial, all on display in this story, also characterize our real-life clothing choices. Our Western culture's refusal to recognize an uncomfortable reality about the clothes we wear carries with it documented threats to personal health and environmental well-being.

Synthetic-fiber clothing is worn with an illusion of safety but hides invisible chemical and other dangers that clothing manufacturers and much of the world's health-care industry ignores, or attempts to rationalize away. The "emperor" that rules most wardrobe choices today is fashion. This emperor is worshipped at an economic altar on which considerations of health and safety have largely been sacrificed.

Only in recent times have humans faced a fashion versus safety dilemma. Ornamenting the human body, whether with paint or tattoos or clothing, seems to have always been our natural impulse, but it was usually a secondary consideration to comfort and protection from the elements. Humankind's earliest clothing may have consisted of leaves and grass matted together and draped around the body, followed later by the use of animal hides to provide protection from sunlight, heat, cold, and the other elements of nature. Some of the earliest sewing needles made from ivory and bone have been carbon-dated to about 30,000BC by archeologists, so we know that for much of human history the production of clothing from animal and plant sources was labor intensive and time consuming.

All of that changed dramatically with the Industrial Revolution of the late eighteenth and early nineteenth centuries, a period in which the textile industry was mechanized so that the mass production of clothing became both possible and profitable. Natural fibers such as cotton, flax, wool, and silk remained the mainstays of this industry until the petrochemical revolution of the twentieth century resulted in the creation of synthetic fibers in chemical laboratories.

Perhaps the most restrictive and unsafe item of clothing introduced in the name of fashion during the nineteenth (or any other) century was the corset. It squeezed women's bodies and crushed their internal organs, even displacing their ribs, until women could hardly breathe or move without experiencing pain. These virtual straitjackets were worn because many women chose to believe these garments made the feminine form more shapely and desirable to men.

There were some notable dissenters to the corset fad and the overall Victorian infatuation with restrictive clothing. A late nineteenth century British group called the Rational Dress Society—whose membership included Mrs. Oscar Wilde, wife of the satirist and writer Oscar Wilde—campaigned against corsets and tight clothing, and advocated the adoption of a style of dress based upon considerations of health.

When it was founded in 1881, the group issued a position statement that could still be used today as a guideline for how to choose safe clothing: "The Rational Dress Society protests against the introduction of any fashion in dress that either deforms the figure, impedes the movements of the body, or in any way tends to injure the health."

Synthetics Displace Natural Fibers

In virtually all areas of life during the twentieth century, synthetics replaced naturally derived consumer products. Nowhere, with the possible exception of cosmetics and personal care products, was this trend more pronounced than in clothing and fabrics manufacturing.

Rayon, introduced in 1924, was the first artificial textile fiber, though variations of this wood-based compound, including cellulose acetate, had been in use since the previous century. But the first truly synthetic fiber was nylon—its petro-molecule source being toluene—whose introduction in 1939 made the mass production of parachutes for use in World War II a less expensive alternative to silk. In that same year, vinyon, a polyvinyl chloride, was created to bind nonwoven fabrics. DuPont chemist Wallace Hume Carothers, generally credited as the inventor of nylon, also probably deserves the title of father of the synthetic textile industry.

Following the creation of nylon, which found its most popular consumer use in women's stockings (panty hose), a series of new synthetics were developed and introduced into mainstream fashion:

- Acrylic and modacrylic in 1950. These "wash-and-wear" fabrics, which often replace wool in sweaters, were considered to be a revolutionary timesaving leap for homemakers, especially those who washed clothes by hand.

- Polyester in 1953. These "wrinkle-free" fabrics, developed from xylene and ethylene, further reduced the amount of clothing made from cotton, particularly men's suits.
- Spandex and olefin in 1959. Sports clothes and bathing suits were the prime uses for stretchable spandex. Sportswear and thermal underwear were made from olefin, which is produced by "cracking" petroleum molecules into propylene and ethylene gases.

The vast majority of clothing items produced in the world today—constituting a $7 trillion a year industry—are either manufactured, or the fabric fibers are grown, using synthetic chemicals, many of which are toxic to human health. As a further challenge to health and safety, most of the cleaning agents used to wash or dry clean clothes contain chemicals that can trigger adverse physical symptoms. These effects on health should be particularly worrisome for parents with babies and young children—who often place clothing in their mouths and then chew and suck on the fabric—because the natural detoxification systems of children's bodies aren't fully developed enough to quickly or completely eliminate fabric chemicals.

According to *The Ecologist* magazine, an estimated eight thousand chemicals are employed to transform raw materials into clothes, a process that involves bleaching, dyeing, scouring, sizing, and finishing the fabrics. Synthetic clothing now commonly contains such toxins as formaldehyde, brominated flame retardants, and perfluorinated chemicals like Teflon fibers to give trousers, skirts, and other apparel "noniron" and "nonwrinkle" durability. (Perfluorinated compounds are classified as cancer-causing agents by the U.S. Environmental Protection Agency guidelines.) Insecticides are even being applied to fibers in the name of protecting health.

The latest clothing craze, which we will detail in chapter 7, takes nanoparticles and adds them to garments, though scientific evidence that these microscopic particles can harm human, animal, and plant life is accumulating.

Health Impacts Are Accumulating

The entire history of synthetic fibers and synthetic clothing amounts to only about six decades of production and use. The era of synthetic clothing really began affecting mainstream wardrobe choices in the 1960s, which means the chemicals used in their production have been in contact with human skin for just a half-century.

Consider what has happened to human health in the industrialized world during that half-century, when synthetic clothing began touching the skin of mainstream consumers. Can it be merely coincidence that, according to the World Health Organization, the industrialized parts of the world have experienced the following:

- Up to one-third of married couples today experience fertility problems.

- Respiratory diseases have increased by 160 percent among preschoolers in Europe and North America.
- Contact dermatitis and other skin ailments have become widespread.
- Our risks of contracting cancer have escalated until one in two males and one in three females will develop this disease in an average lifetime.
- If you're a woman, you now have a one-in-eight chance of developing breast cancer in an average lifetime. For postmenopausal women, the rate of breast cancer has escalated by 22 percent over just the past three decades.

Our own experience with the three hundred thousand guests who have visited The Hippocrates Health Institute over the years bears out these statistics. Once natural-fiber clothing began to be replaced by synthetics in the 1970s, we started seeing increasing numbers of guests showing up with breast cancer, prostate cancer, and a range of allergic conditions. That trend has accelerated with each passing decade as natural-fiber clothing disappeared from store shelves. It became apparent to us at Hippocrates that the addition of chemical clothing to underlying chemical problems already existing in the body creates even more chronic and serious health problems.

Human-made petrochemical fibers restrict and suffocate the skin, our largest and most sensitive body organ, making it unable to breathe properly so it can release toxins. Most people don't realize that our skin is our body's most important eliminative organ. By some estimates, we release a pound of toxins every day through our skin, assuming that it's allowed to vent as nature intended. If we hold back any percentage of these toxins from being released, they accumulate in body fat and body organs to become like a time bomb, primed to detonate as some future health malady.

Many of the impacts on health from chemicals used in synthetic clothing are being documented in medical journal studies, but these reports rarely receive mainstream media attention. To give just one illustration, contact dermatitis and other allergenic effects caused by skin exposure to synthetic clothing "is not only more frequent than previously thought," according to a 2003 study in the medical journal *Dermatology Online,* "but is also increasing." This probably comes as news to you because that study, like so many others dealing with the health consequences of synthetic clothing, failed to receive the public attention it deserved due to the "Emperor's New Clothes syndrome," that wall of silence and denial surrounding the fashion manufacturing industry.

In *Killer Clothes,* that wall of silence will be breached as we reveal the many ways that synthetic clothing, chemicals added to garments, and tight clothing and tight shoes create acute problems for human health. Here are just a few examples of our findings:

- Medical evidence has emerged that the longer a woman wears a bra, especially a tight one, the greater her chance of developing breast problems, including breast cancer.

- Synthetic fibers pose such a fire and burn hazard that the U.S. Marine Corps prohibits its troops in Iraq from wearing synthetic clothing while off base.
- Medical studies have found that synthetic fibers help to induce muscle fatigue and muscle motor disorders, which for competitive athletes can mean the difference between winning and losing.
- Studies have determined that synthetic fibers produce electrostatic discharges and, as a result, the wearing of tight synthetic clothing and undergarments contributes to infertility in men.
- Permethrin is being added to civilian outdoor wear and military uniforms even though no tests have been conducted of this insecticide's long-term impact on human health.
- Silver particles called nanosilver are being applied to name-brand clothing lines as antiodor, antiwrinkle, and antistain agents, though medical studies raise serious doubts about their safety.

Clothing manufacturers and even many toxicologists choose to believe that absorbing tiny amounts of toxic chemicals from individual items of clothing cannot be harmful to you. That often-repeated argument will be addressed in this book in several different ways.

First, we don't just absorb synthetic chemicals one at a time during the average day. We are exposed to hundreds of chemicals as a result of using a wide array of consumer products on our skin that contain synthetic ingredients, particularly cosmetics and personal care products. Many of these same chemicals are used in synthetic clothing. That means we absorb tiny amounts of chemicals repeatedly from multiple sources until they add up and reach a tipping point within us that could be harmful.

Second, the rationalization that "the toxin levels are too small to inflict harm," as repeated by representatives of the synthetic clothing industry, fails to take into account the role of chemical synergies and their impact on health. While some individual chemicals alone may not endanger your health, when chemicals from multiple sources combine and interact inside of your body, they can have unpredictable and potentially powerful effects with health consequences. These synergistic processes constitute the "black hole" of ignorance within the fields of toxicology and preventive medicine.

A Return to Safe Clothing

Is it too much to expect that the clothing we allow to touch our skin should be as natural and safe as it can possibly be? Shouldn't we be as concerned about wearing toxic chemicals as we are about ingesting or inhaling toxins?

Our freedom to choose and wear natural versus synthetic clothing has narrowed over the past few decades because the lower costs of synthetics have crowded natural fibers out of the marketplace. That's why the United Nations Food and Agriculture Organization declared 2009 to be the International Year of Natural Fibres. The need to revive and promote the sustainability of natural clothing industries worldwide came about because, as the U.N. group declared on its website, the natural fibers industry "has lost a lot of its market share due to the increased use of synthetic fibers."

But as we will explain in this book, all of us retain the power to minimize risks to our health by taking simple precautions and practicing mindfulness about our clothing choices and the buying options that we still have. *Killer Clothes* will help to guide you in making those important decisions by presenting lists of safe products and safety-conscious manufacturers that still value consumer health over easy profits.

Killer Clothes also documents how synthetic clothing impacts much more than just our personal health and well-being. Chemical clothing affects the health of the entire planet, from the toxic production methods used, to the chemicals employed in the cleaning of these items, to clothing disposal practices that allow these nonbiodegradable products to continue to harm the environment long after their users have ceased to exist.

German chemist Michael Braungart and American architect William McDonough, authors of the 2002 book on ecologically intelligent design, *Cradle to Cradle: Remaking the Way We Make Things,* described how "textiles are quite literally woven into the fabric of life," but our reliance on dangerous synthetics has steered us into a toxic blind alley. "The industry that launched the Industrial Revolution has long illustrated some of its most notorious design failures," they wrote. "About one half of the world's wastewater problems are linked to the production of textile goods, and many of the chemicals used to dye and finish fabrics are known to harm human health."

"Often, the clippings from fabric mills are so loaded with dangerous chemicals they are handled like toxic waste," Braungart and McDonough point out, "while the products made from these materials are considered safe for use in the home." The same troubling double standard holds true for all synthetic clothing—the dangerous chemicals used to produce them are considered toxic by manufacturers and public health institutions, but the clothing produced with these chemicals is treated as safe for use on human skin.

The choices we face as consumers and stewards of the Earth should be stark and clear. Organically grown natural fibers pose few threats to human health, whereas chemical fibers and synthetic clothing contribute to a long list of documented human ailments and degenerative conditions for the planet. Energy for the production of natural fibers comes from the sun, a renewable resource, whereas energy used to produce synthetic fibers comes mostly from fossil fuels, which generate multiple types of environmental pollutants that help to accelerate global warming.

You've heard it said that we become what we eat. If so, then we also become what we choose to wear! With synthetic clothing, we literally absorb some of the chemicals used in their manufacture. Safe clothes made from natural organic fibers, by contrast, help to produce healthy bodies and healthy minds.

It is our hope that you will find this book to be a useful resource that will help you to navigate this toxic minefield. Together we can build a healthier future for all.

CHAPTER 1

Tight Clothing's Link to Health Problems

Bras May Be a Breast Cancer Trigger

What if everything you thought you knew about bras and breast cancer turned out to be wrong? Can you question your long-held assumptions and personal habits, but more importantly, make necessary lifestyle corrections that will protect and improve your health? Is putting your "chest eggs in a tight nest," as breasts in bras are sometimes equated, really necessary or even healthy?

These are the kinds of questions that Dr. Elizabeth R. Vaughan began asking herself and her patients over a decade ago. Her background and upbringing isn't that of someone who might ordinarily be expected to become a maverick health-care provider, much less one who challenges conventional health wisdom with passionate conviction. She's the daughter of two physicians, a descendant of four generations of physicians, and her great-grandfather was president of the American Medical Association. But her provocative outside-the-mainstream ideas about bras, toxins, and breast cancer prompted *USA Today* to call her "the Erin Brockovich of medicine." You might recall

Erin Brockovich as the legal crusader who defied conventional wisdom and exposed the toxic contamination of an entire town, and whose story was later told in a movie starring Julia Roberts.

What Dr. Vaughan, CEO of Vaughan Medical Center in Greensboro, North Carolina, began to notice was a relationship between the development of breast lumps and cysts and the wearing of bras. She personally treated more than one hundred women who, in her words, "chose to go bra free after yet another biopsy of a lump in their breasts or aspiration of a cyst. Over three to six months, their breast cysts and lumps got smaller and less tender, and they developed no new lumps that we could detect." Dr. Vaughan's observation has since been demonstrated in practice by other health-care providers.

Breast cysts may be one of the flashing red warning signs for the onset of breast cancer. A 1999 study in the prestigious British medical journal *The Lancet* examined 1,374 women with breast cysts and tracked them based on their incidence of breast cancer. It was found that premenopausal women with breast cysts had a nearly six-fold increased risk of breast cancer compared to women who didn't have breast cysts. Here is how the authors of this study succinctly summarized their findings: "Women with breast cysts are at an increased risk of breast cancer."

That shouldn't come as a surprise given that most women wear bras that are much too tight for them and have worn them this way since they received their first training bra as a young girl. According to the Johns Hopkins Breast Center, "as many as 80 percent of women are actually wearing a bra that is the wrong size for them," a chronic condition that can produce health problems, particularly in the backs of women with large breasts.

With a connection possibly established between breast cysts and breast cancer, along with Dr. Vaughan's findings that bras cause or exacerbate the development of breast cysts, you don't need to be the Sherlock Holmes of common sense to grasp that bras, lymphatic drainage impairment, breast cysts, and breast cancer may be linked, much like a chain reaction automobile wreck. A key circumstantial piece of evidence showing a link between bras and breast cancer emerged in 1991 from a study of breast size and breast cancer risk by researchers in the Department of Epidemiology at the Harvard School of Public Health. Published in the *European Journal of Cancer,* this survey of thousands of women found that "Premenopausal women who do not wear bras had half the risk of breast cancer compared to bra users."

The study authors speculated that this could be because these premenopausal women are "thinner and likely to have smaller breasts." But that observation received little or no support from subsequent medical studies. As the director of the Johns Hopkins Breast Center declared in 2007: "Simply having breasts and being female places all women at risk.

Women with size 32AA bras get breast cancer just like someone with 46DDs."

This Harvard study finding about bra usage and a higher risk for breast cancer should have set off alarm bells within the health field and the clothing industry. At the very least, it should have spawned a spate of new studies exploring this connection between bra use and breast cancer. But it caused barely a ripple in public health awareness. Once again, as in the "Emperor's New Suit," reflexive rejection and obstinate denial triumphed over reality and common sense.

More Evidence Accumulates

Medical Anthropologist Sydney Ross Singer began to notice that when his wife removed her bra, both of her breasts were "outlined by dark red lines, marking the areas around her breasts and over her shoulders. The lines had been left by her bra." This observation came in the wake of his wife's discovery in 1991 that she had a suspicious lump on her breast. Their search for medical answers gave rise to a series of questions that in turn spawned a theory—could the constrictive nature of the brassiere have suppressed her lymphatic system, the internal network of blood vessels that flushes toxins from the breasts and other parts of the body? Can toxins accumulate in breast tissue as a result of this constriction, and can that accumulation in turn trigger the growth of breast lumps and even the onset of breast cancer?

To test their theory, Singer and his wife designed and carried out a Bra and Breast Cancer Study of 4,700 women, ages thirty to seventy-nine, who were interviewed in five U.S. cities—New York, Dallas, Phoenix, Denver, and San Francisco. About half had been diagnosed with breast cancer, the other half had no breast cancer diagnosis. The questions asked of each woman included: Does your bra ever leave red marks on your skin or cause irritation? How long do you wear your bra each day on the average? During what stages in your teenage and adult life did you not wear a bra?

Striking differences emerged in the answers given by the breast cancer and noncancer groups regarding bra usage and bra comfort. Only 1 percent of the cancer group wore their bras for fewer than twelve hours a day, compared to 20 percent of the noncancer group, who wore bras fewer than twelve hours a day. Eighteen percent of the cancer group wore their bras to bed, compared to just 3 percent of the noncancer group. There were other statistically significant differences between the two groups. Only 4 percent of the cancer group had breast-fed their children, for instance, compared to 14 percent of the noncancer group. Almost zero percent of breast cancer victims regularly went braless before their diagnosis, versus 5 percent of women in the noncancer group who regularly went without bras.

Here is how Singer calculated the cancer risks from bras based on the study results:

- There is a six-fold greater incidence of breast cancer among women who wear a bra all day and to bed than among the general population.
- Going braless results in twenty-one-fold reduction in breast cancer.
- Breast-feeding affords three and one-half times the protection against breast cancer. One reason may be that breast-feeding stimulates greater drainage within the lymphatic system of the breasts, helping to prevent the accumulation of toxins. This observation is in line with other study findings that women who have never given birth have a higher incidence of breast cancer.

Though not proving a link between bra usage and breast cancer, this study nonetheless produced evidence suggesting that Singer's theory could have merit. "Breast cancer may be caused by the combined effects of toxins and bras on breasts," Singer concluded in the book *Dressed to Kill: The Link Between Breast Cancer and Bras.* "Bras are not the cause of breast cancer, but they may be a trigger for it."

Other circumstantial support for Singer's theory comes from cultural observations made in the book *Cancer on Five Continents,* published by the International Association of Cancer Registries in France. Women with the lowest incidence of breast cancer live in cultures where bras are not part of traditional wardrobes. These cultures include populations in parts of India, Israel, and Singapore, as well as some American Indian tribal groups.

As a follow-up to their U.S. study, Singer and his wife did a survey of bra use and breast cancer in Fiji, where an estimated half of all women adhere to cultural tradition and refuse to wear Western-style bras. A Fijian health ministry official told the couple that their bra and breast cancer theory made sense because "our working women are now getting breast cancer. They are the ones who wear bras." The Singers examined several dozen case histories of breast cancer among Fijian women, and every woman turned out to have broken from cultural norms to become a bra wearer. "We found that, given women from the same village (genetically related), with the same diet, the ones who developed breast cancer were the ones who wore bras," reported Singer and Grismaijer in 2007.

Mainstream practitioners of Western medicine continue to reject the idea of any possible connection between bras and the occurrence of breast cancer. They do so, for the most part, reflexively, without ever having examined the evidence.

Dr. Marissa Weiss, writing in *Prevention* magazine, made this bold claim without citing any medical studies: "It's not true that wearing a bra, especially underwire bras, traps toxins by limiting lymph and blood flow in your breasts, increasing risk." A similar claim, once again without supporting medical documentation, was made by Lillie

Shockney, Administrative Director of the Johns Hopkins Breast Center (funded by the Avon Foundation), who wrote in her December 16, 2008, health column for Yahoo.com: "This is a myth that needs to finally be put to rest. Having a bra that is too tight, too small, underwired, or filled with air pockets or water doesn't contribute to someone developing breast cancer." Shockney's column drew numerous responses from readers on Yahoo who challenged her with the same question: How do you know?

Other Medical Research Linking Bras and Disease

The heavier her bra material, the hotter a woman's breasts become, and this elevated breast temperature may contribute to the onset of breast cancer. This was the conclusion of a 1978 study in *The Lancet* by Dr. John M. Douglass of Los Angeles. He based his conclusions on examining several hundred women in his medical practice.

Bras increase breast pain and discomfort, but when women discontinue wearing bras, the pain decreases or disappears. Two British breast surgeons, Dr. Simon Cawthorne of Frenchay Hospital in Bristol, England, and Dr. Robert Mansel of the University of Wales Medical School, studied one hundred women for three months to see if going bra free lessened breast pain. The findings were conclusive—a majority of premenopausal women did improve their breast health and comfort as a result of going bra free.

Pressure on the breasts from bras can elevate the core temperature of the body and suppress the production of melatonin, an important antioxidant for immune system health. Melatonin also has anti-cancer properties that are useful in preventing breast cancer. In 2000 that was the finding of two researchers at Japan's Nara Women's University who studied and measured the sleep-wake cycles of ten women, aged eighteen to twenty-three, to document the effect of bras on body temperature and melatonin levels.

In 2002 six other Japanese researchers did a study that documented how skin pressure as a result of wearing bras affects the autonomic nervous system in a harmful way. "Our data indicate," wrote the researchers in the *Journal of Physiological Anthropology and Applied Human Science,* "that the higher clothing pressures exerted by a conventional brassiere have a significant negative impact on the autonomic nervous system activity, which is predominantly attributable to the significant decrease in the parasympathetic as well as the thermoregulatory sympathetic nerve activities. Since the autonomic nervous system activity plays an important role in modulating the internal environment in the human body, excess clothing pressures caused by constricting types of foundation garments on the body would consequently undermine women's health."

Beginning in 1967 a series of studies in the *Journal of the American Medical Association* and elsewhere documented how bras that are manufactured with spandex fibers can cause skin problems in some bra wearers due to contact with the chemicals used in the production process that remain in the garments.

Meet The Breast Toxins

Breast cancer specialists are in general agreement that about 85 percent of the two-hundred thousand women in the United States who are diagnosed with the disease each year have no inherited genetic predisposition, which means that unhealthful lifestyle choices and the absorption of environmental pollutants account for the vast majority of breast cancer cases.

Many health-care professionals fail to take into account that human skin, the body's largest organ, acts as a highly absorbent carrier for chemicals that come into direct contact with our body's "miracle garment," as skin is often called. Common chemicals that can regularly come into contact with your skin and be absorbed by body tissues include the ingredients in cosmetics and personal care products, as well as chemicals used in the manufacture of synthetic clothing.

When toxins enter the body through the mouth and end up in the intestines, they are channeled by the blood into the liver, where detoxification naturally occurs. When toxins are absorbed through the skin, however, they bypass the liver. In fact, as toxicology specialist Dr. Samuel Epstein states in his 2009 book, *Toxic Beauty,* about toxins in cosmetics and personal care products, medical evidence exists that human skin is even more permeable than the nutrient-absorbing intestines, which makes skin the primary way that toxins invade the body. "As difficult as it might be to believe," wrote Dr. Epstein, a professor emeritus at the University of Illinois and founder of the Cancer Prevention Coalition, "mainstream manufacturers and regulatory authorities appear unaware of the high permeability of skin, or else simply choose to ignore this as a critical concern."

The list of possible chemicals that could be accumulating in women's breasts as a result of their skin exposure to everyday products and clothing is a lengthy one. Let's start with preservatives called parabens that are found in deodorants and antiperspirants and have been incriminated as a probable cause of breast cancer.

A 2004 study in the *Journal of Applied Toxicology* examined concentrations of parabens in human breast tumors and found a high correlation. As Dr. Epstein commented, "Parabens' presence in breast tissue on its own incriminates them as a possible cause of breast cancer, but they have also been shown to stimulate the growth of estrogen-sensitive breast cancer cells in laboratory tests."

Triclosan is a second type of personal care product preservative that has been shown in laboratory tests to induce hormone disruptive effects that could trigger breast cancer. Triclosan is often found in antibacterial soaps, deodorants, and other consumer goods, but most alarming, it's also increasingly being added to synthetic clothing to prevent bacterial growth. Surveys conducted by Greenpeace International and other environmental and consumer groups have detected triclosan in a high percentage of umbilical cord blood samples and in the breast milk of half of all women that the groups tested, so we know this chemical bioaccumulates in the body easily and persists in the body over time.

Detergents, called surfactants, appear in consumer products as cleansers but also are used in the production of textiles and clothing. One of these detergents, a nonoxynol known as 4-NP, has been lab tested in animals and found to trigger the development of breast cancer. A 1994 study published in the medical journal *Endocrinology* concluded: "Long-term exposure to 4-NP could leave individuals at a significantly increased risk of developing breast cancer." This chemical and some other related surfactants have been banned or severely limited from use in the production of clothing by the government of Norway out of concern for the impact on human health, yet these chemicals are still commonly used in the United States and most of the rest of the world.

Or consider the role played by the ingredients in most brand-name shampoos. A carcinogen called 1,4-dioxane, which is readily absorbed through the skin, contaminates an entire category of ethoxylate detergents—any with "eth" in their names, such as myreth and oleth—and this contaminant was listed in the medical journal *Cancer'* s 2007 review of carcinogens as a producer of breast cancer in rodent testing. In February 2007 a *Los Angeles Times* article reported that eighteen personal care products tested by an independent laboratory found high levels of dioxane.

Still another concern for women should be the ingredients in brand-name antiperspirants. A 2006 study published in the *Journal of Applied Toxicology* found evidence that aluminum chloride, used in high concentrations in most antiperspirants, is a hormone disruptive chemical that could trigger the onset of breast cancer. Study author Philippa Darbre, PhD, expressed concern that aluminum chloride in antiperspirants is absorbed through the underarms and can accumulate in the adjoining breast tissue. Professor Darbre also brought up the issue of chemical synergies from multiple chemicals in personal care products acting together inside the body. "Each of these agents on their own may not have a powerful effect," she wrote, "but we need to see what happens when a number of them act together. It could be that this would have a significant effect on diseases like breast cancer."

Lymph System Is Key in Toxin Removal

As women absorb the chemicals mentioned above from skin contact with consumer products and synthetic clothing, the toxins accumulate in breast tissue, so the theory goes, and remain there because constrictive bra use prevents the breast's lymphatic system from draining properly. That could be one of the triggers for the development of breast cancer. Consider how there are three primary steps or stages to this theory.

Step one, toxins that can cause cancer, such as those in consumer products, are absorbed by the body. They then accumulate in fat tissue because fat tissue attracts toxins like a magnet. A woman's breast tissue is mostly composed of fat cells, so toxins tend to be stored there.

Step two, the body's lymph system plays a role, along with the liver, in removing toxins. If the lymph system fails to play its designated role effectively, toxins get stored in fat cells for too long, and that triggers the development of cancer cells.

Step three, because your body's lymph system is reliant on passive forms of fluid propulsion like movement and exercise (unlike your heart, which drives blood through your vessels), the lymph system is sensitive to outside physical pressure. Since there are lymph pathways and lymph nodes in your armpits, under your breasts, and between your breasts, a tight-fitting bra can squeeze those areas and prevent proper drainage of lymph fluid that might ordinarily carry away toxins stored in fat cells.

If you're a woman, the next time you remove your bra after a day of use, try standing in front of a mirror and note the position of the strap marks. (If you're a man, take note of these marks on your wife or significant other.) The more your bra was designed to mold your breasts into a particular shape, the more apparent these strap marks will be. This is visual evidence of how breast constriction interrupts drainage from the lymphatic system of your breast tissue. Add to this constriction and immobilization an elevation in breast temperature, especially on hot days, combined with extended bra use, and guess what may happen? Your stored stew of toxins gets cooked inside of you.

On the website www.breastnotes.com, the relationship between the constrictions of breasts inside bras and the impairment of lymphatic drainage is addressed this way: "Unsupported breasts (of any size) will most likely move when the woman is walking or moving about. This is a natural movement, and there seems to be a reason for it. We have breast massage articles from several experts that address the question of breast movement and its relationship to the natural flow of lymphatic fluids in the breasts. Since there is no 'heart' to move the lymphatic fluid, we must rely on body movement and muscular contractions to move the fluid."

More Skin Problems Caused by Bras

Hundreds, if not thousands, of women began complaining in 2008 that their bras were creating serious rashes and even scarring of the skin on and around their breasts.

"My bra kept me burning and itching and gave me a horrible rash," reported sixty-six-year-old Jerilyn Amaya of West Palm Beach, Florida. "I finally stopped wearing the bra and the symptoms disappeared."

Ms. Amaya and more than six hundred other women across the United States joined in federal lawsuits filed in Florida, New Jersey, and New York against Victoria's Secret and its parent company, Limited Brands Inc., accusing the manufacturer of "negligently designing undergarments and misrepresenting the safety" of their products. Specifically, the lawsuits alleged that Victoria's Secret bras contained formaldehyde resins at levels harmful to human health.

When the bras are heated in a clothes dryer, according to the lawsuits, formaldehyde embedded in the fabric of the bras is released. Toxicologist Patricia Williams told the Associated Press in April 2009 that "this is not a little clothing rash" caused by the bras. She said, "The extent and severity of it is just unbelievable. Many of (the plaintiffs) have scars that seem to be permanent."

A spokesperson for Limited Brands replied that testing of their bras showed "only small traces" of formaldehyde that "wouldn't cause any health problems." Furthermore, said the spokesperson, the company doesn't intentionally add formaldehyde to its bras.

At least two medical studies can be cited as offering some support for the crucial role that your lymphatic system plays in preventing, lessening, or triggering breast cancer. In a December 2002 issue of the medical journal *Lymphology,* researchers presented study findings showing how normal breast lymph drainage is an important predictor of whether a woman with breast cancer will survive. If a breast cancer patient's lymph vessels are obstructed, her chances of survival were rated as poor, whereas women with normal breast lymph drainage had a 30 percent higher survival rate.

The second study was conducted in Britain and was summarized this way in an October 31, 2000, edition of the *Sunday Telegraph (London):* "Wearing a bra exposes women to a 'statistically significant' risk of increased breast pain, cysts in the breast and might even be linked to the development of cancer." One hundred women who regularly suffered from breast pain or breast cysts were asked to go bra free for three months. A significant number reported a reduction in their symptoms during this period. The newspaper further reported that the scientists in this study "suspect problems are caused by bras suppressing the lymphatic system—the network of vessels that flushes toxic waste from the body. Professor Robert Mansel, a professor of surgery at the University Hospital of Wales, said the garments appear to be compressing the body at the outer upper part of the breast—the area where 80 percent of the lymph flows." This study was considered particularly important in Britain because an estimated 40 percent of women in that country complain of breast pain and breast cysts.

Breast-feeding provides a form of insurance against breast cancer by helping to stimulate lymphatic system circulation within breast tissue. A breast-feeding advocacy group, La Leche League International, compiled a list of medical studies on its website, www.llli.org, that supports this point of view. Here are a few representative examples of those study findings:

- About 1,432 new cases of breast cancer each year in the state of California are attributable to women having never breast-fed their babies, and a simple lifestyle change of breast-feeding, or lengthening the duration of breast-feeding, could prevent many cases of breast cancer, according to a June 27, 2006, study article in the journal *BMC Cancer.*

- Longer duration of breast-feeding could "reduce breast cancer risk significantly," according to a German study of 706 breast cancer cases, published in February 2003 in the *International Journal of Epidemiology.*
- The incidence of breast cancer among women in developed countries could be reduced by half, from 6.3 to 2.7 cases per hundred women, if breast-feeding today were as common as a century ago, and the longer a woman breast-feeds, the more protection against breast cancer she is afforded, concluded a July 20, 2002, study published in *The Lancet.*
- Finally, a 2001 article in the *American Journal of Epidemiology,* titled "Long-term Breastfeeding Lowers Mother's Breast Cancer Risk," determined that women who breast-fed a child for more than two years had a 54 percent reduced risk of developing breast cancer compared with women who breast-fed for fewer than six months. This protective effect was found to exist both before and after the onset of menopause.

What Have You Sacrificed for Fashion?

Most women who we come into contact with on a daily basis share this experience and opinion of bras—they are uncomfortable, they unnecessarily restrict movement and blood flow, they impede our skin's ability to breathe and release toxins, and instinctively we know that bras and the bra industry are doing harm to women's bodies. So why do women wear them?

Brassieres are a relatively recent development in the history of women's clothing, having been patented in 1914 by Mary Phelps Jacobs to be an alternative to the corsets that had contorted and restricted women from the waist to chest ever since they first became popular during the 1500s in Europe.

Breast Massage Helps Remove Toxins

Lymphatic drainage massage (LDM) is a manual technique that you can perform on your own to help keep your breasts free of cysts, lumps, and cancer.

While any form of massage to the breasts may assist lymphatic flow, LDM differs from regular therapeutic massage in several respects. The strokes of your hand on your breast should be light and superficial in LDM, should be performed slowly, and should manipulate the breasts in alternating clockwise and counter-clockwise directions for the maximum and most beneficial fluid release.

Because bras lift and shape the breasts upward in sometimes provocative ways, our culture came to view them as a kind of sexual garment. Hollywood in the 1940s and '50s used movie icon Jayne Mansfield and other starlets to further market bras as sex appeal enhancers. That public perception of sexuality contributed to bras becoming the wearer's statement of style and fashion, irrespective of whether the undergarments served any real practical function.

So what do bras actually do that is useful? Answers provided by habitual bra wearers and the bra manufacturing industry range from "keeping breasts from sagging" to "making breasts appear more modest when in public." Let's address these reasons and concerns one by one with counterarguments provided by independent-minded women and medical authorities who have taken the time to study the subject of bras and breasts.

Do bras really keep breasts from sagging? Three medical researchers at the Otsuma Women's University in Tokyo, Japan, conducted a 1990 experiment in which eleven women, aged twenty-two to thirty-nine, wore bras for three months and then, for another three months, they went without bras. Measurements and photographs were taken once a week throughout the six-month experiment.

Here are the key findings of this experiment, as described in a medical journal (Ashizawa 1990): "In all subjects, after three months of brassiere constraint, the underbust circumference was smaller but the chest circumference became enlarged, the distance between the right and left nipples became wider, and the breasts tended to hang down. This change was more marked in obese subjects with pendent breasts. And when this type of subject wore a 'well-fitted' brassiere for a long time, her breast form became developed, that is, her breasts hung down more."

Ligaments in a woman's breasts hold the breasts up and in place. The more a woman wears a bra, the more those ligaments atrophy, getting weaker and smaller. The longer a woman goes braless, the more those ligaments strengthen over time. That is why some women experience soreness in their breasts when they go braless—the ligaments have weakened from lack of use. These are just basic facts of human physiology.

Dr. Susan M. Love, in *Dr. Susan Love's Breast Book,* called the belief that the breasts need to be supported a prevalent and persistent myth. "Wearing a bra has no medical necessity whatsoever," she declared. "The decision to wear or not wear one is purely aesthetic, or emotional."

In their book, *The Complete Book of Breast Care,* Dr. Niels H. Lauersen and Eileen Stukane made a similar point: "Is a bra good or bad for your breasts? Neither! There is no medical reason to wear a bra, so the decision is yours, based on your own personal comfort and aesthetics. Whether you have always worn a bra or always gone braless, age and breast-feeding will naturally cause your breasts to sag."

Dr. Christiane Northrup of the University of Vermont College of Medicine, and author of *Women's Bodies, Women's Wisdom,* cautions bra wearers: "Stop wearing an underwire bra. Too often this kind of bra cuts off circulation of both blood and lymph fluid around the breast, chest wall, and surrounding tissue."

To err on the side of caution concerning your breast health, it's best that you don't wear a bra at all. But if you do wear one, limit your bra usage to only those absolutely necessary occasions. That might include when you exercise, jog in public, or go to the gym. Find a sports bra that gives you the breast support that you think you want and need without being overly restrictive. And if you do wear a bra to work or during the day, *never ever* wear it to bed. The more time you spend wearing a bra, the higher your risk of developing serious problems with your breasts.

Breast Cancer Risk Is Increased by Acrylic and Nylon

If you repeatedly absorb chemicals from certain fibers at an early age, you run a risk of contracting a variety of diseases and ailments. The latest evidence to emerge about the lifelong consequences of chemical contact is in relation to exposure to acrylic and nylon fibers and how they multiply the risk of breast cancer later in life.

As part of ongoing research to understand the role of synthetic chemicals in the development of breast cancer, a team of Canadian scientists and chemists from Montreal examined the exposure of 1,169 post-menopausal women to about three hundred chemical substances. What they found and reported in 2010 should alarm any woman who has had sustained contact, especially in an occupational setting, with nylon or acrylic fabrics.

Of the three hundred substances that were analyzed in this epidemiological study, exposure to acrylics and nylon demonstrated the greatest association with breast cancer in women fifty to seventy-five years of age. These risks peaked for exposures before the age of thirty-six and increased with each additional decade of exposure.

The actual increase in breast cancer risk from exposure to the chemicals in each fabric is quite substantial. Women exposed to acrylic fibers early in life multiplied their breast cancer risk by sevenfold, while nylon fiber exposure almost doubled their risk, according to 2010 study results reported in the British medical journal *Occupational and Environmental Medicine.* Acrylic synthetic fibers are derived from acrylic acid. It is used in clothing as a less expensive alternative to cashmere. Acrylic doesn't dye well, so its polymers are dyed before it becomes fiber or fabric. Static buildup is a common problem with this fabric, and it is known to irritate people with sensitive skin.

Nylon is formed from a reaction of diamine and dicarboxylic acid Acetic acid and other chemicals are added during the production process. Originally invented as a silk replacement, nylon became popular in the 1940s for use in women's stockings.

It is also found in a wide variety of other fabrics, from bridal veils to vests.

While the scientists involved in this study conceded their results might be due to chance, at least until other studies replicate and expand on their findings, they pointed out that the association they found was consistent with many other studies showing the sensitivity of breast tissue to chemicals. If the breast tissue exposure to chemicals occurs when breast cells remain active, which is into the forties for most women, chemical contact can be particularly powerful in creating toxic consequences later in life.

Tight Shoes Are Not a Fashion Requirement

No matter what materials your shoes happen to be made from, they count as a form of clothing apparel. Like other articles of clothing, shoes come manufactured with many of the chemicals that make clothing so problematic to health.

Shoes made in part or whole from petrochemicals generate many of the same health and environmental hazards as synthetic clothing. One clear impact on ecosystems is that shoes don't easily (if at all) biodegrade once discarded in landfills.

Seven Bra-Free Options for Breast Health

You can appear in public bra free without having to feel self-conscious that you're being stared at or that you're in violation of a workplace dress code. Here are seven simple and inexpensive options for bra-free breast health.

1. Wear a sleeveless undershirt. Most often sold as men's wear, these undershirts are comfortable and come in a variety of thicknesses.

2. Wear a camisole. Whether silk or cotton, these garments have adjustable clasps and give the appearance of a bra to observers.

3. Wear a vest. Either a men's or women's dress or casual vest can be worn over your blouse to hide the outline of your breasts.

4. Wear a loosely fitted top. Depending on your breast size, loose tops can camouflage your breasts effectively.

5. Wear a shirt with pockets. Pockets camouflage the outline of your breasts and nipples.

6. Wear a bust-free bra. These are two cups that cling inside your outer garment's fabric.

7. Wear NuBra cups. Check out www.nubra.com for examples of adhesive cups that can cover your breasts to keep your nipples from showing through outer clothing.

Consider the effects of just one chemical used in the production of one type of shoe—those made of leather. Up until the mid- to late twentieth century, vegetable chemicals were used to tan leather to prepare it to be made into shoes. Chromium tanning replaced vegetable tanning because manufacturers found it to be a cheaper and faster process.

Chromium can be a carcinogen, and because most shoes today are made in developing countries with almost nonexistent safety and environmental rules, chromium contamination of people and ecosystems is disturbingly common. As William McDonough and Michael Braungart observe in their book, *Cradle to Cradle,* another problem with the use of chromium in shoe production comes "when manufacturing wastes are dumped into nearby bodies of water or incinerated, either of which distributes toxins."

These two authors also point out how rubber-soled shoes usually contain lead and plastics, and that as the shoes are worn, "particles degrade into the atmosphere and soil. It cannot be safely consumed, either by you or by the environment."

Foot Health Is Often Overlooked

Many people unnecessarily sacrifice comfort and their foot health in pursuit of some trendy designer's idea of which shoes should be fashionable to wear in public. A vast majority of foot problems are the result of incorrect or poorly chosen footwear, according to Britain's Society of Chiropodists and Podiatrists, which did a survey of two thousand people in 2009 that found four in ten women purchase and then wear uncomfortable shoes because they are considered fashionable. By contrast, about 17 percent of the men surveyed admitted to intentionally buying shoes in an incorrect size because of how they look when worn.

Four common foot problems caused by poor shoe choices—conditions experienced by 80 percent of the women surveyed—include:

- blisters created by the friction from ill-fitting shoes
- corns caused by rubbing and pressure
- bunions in which foot compression creates painful swelling on the sides of the big toes

A Tight-Fitting Clothes Infection Warning for Women

You may think those tight-fitting jeans and short skirts make you look and feel sexy, but would you still wear them if the unexpected price you had to pay was a serious vaginal infection?

A 1983 study in the *American Journal of Public Health* examined 160 women and divided them into two equal groups—one that primarily wore tight-fitting garments 80 percent or more of the time, and one that primarily wore loose clothes 80 percent or more of the time. The results were clear.

"Our present study confirms our previous observation," wrote the study authors, "that wearing of tight fitting clothing, coupled with nylon underwear and/or panty hose, creates more warmth and moisture in the vaginal and cervical areas, thus producing an environment favorable for colonization of *Candida albicans* and other yeasts."

- ingrown toenails produced by tight footwear, especially when exacerbated by tight socks

A second survey by the same foot organization, this time questioning one thousand pregnant women in June 2010, found even more health problems associated with wearing the wrong size shoes in the name of fashion. Many of these women wore ballet pumps (53 percent), or flip-flops (66 percent), and even high heels (32 percent) during the nine months of their pregnancies.

Seven out of every ten pregnant women reported problems with their feet from these poor shoe choices. Swollen ankles turned out to be a complaint confessed by 37 percent of those questioned, 45 percent had swollen feet, and 16 percent described acute arch and heel pain.

One might think it would be a matter of common sense that pregnancy confers the need to take special precautions concerning all aspects of health. But suffering in order to be seen as remaining fashionable is an old habit that too few women consider while pregnant. The effects of weight gain and hormonal changes are exacerbated by wearing shoes that offer little or no body support. High heels are particularly unsafe, not only shortening calf muscles, but also increasing pressure on the back and knees, which are all conditions that increase the wearer's prospect of experiencing dangerous falls.

Don't Forget Those Flip-Flops

They are usually loose on your feet, and they've been worn by humans for thousands of years—the Egyptian King Tutankhamen and Queen Cleopatra used them—but that doesn't mean flip-flop sandals are good for your feet, especially if you wear them frequently.

"If you wear them all the time, they aren't good for you," claims Dr. Kathya Zinszer, associate professor of podiatric medicine at Temple's School of Podiatric Medicine. "They give you no support and they don't protect your feet."

Research studies support her point of view. A 2008 Auburn University study documented that people who wear flip-flops take shorter steps, and the heels of their feet hit the ground with less vertical force than when they wear other shoes. The cumulative impact of this repeated motion is pain in the wearer's ankles, feet, and legs.

Flip-flop wearers seem willing to sacrifice foot health for temporary comfort, at least until the pain gets too severe and they begin to realize its source. If you experience foot problems, start wearing a more structured shoe that protects the feet and ankles.

Always keep in mind that if your feet hurt, no matter what kind of shoe you are wearing, something is wrong and needs to be corrected. You may need to make some overdue changes in your footwear and perhaps even in your ideas about what is stylish.

CHAPTER 2

Chemical Clothes Surround Us

Take an inventory of your wardrobe. Start with the labels to determine what percentage of your clothing is synthetic. This will become your risk-to-reward ratio. The more synthetic clothing you have, the greater your risk of absorbing enough toxic chemicals to affect your health.

In this section you will learn what fabrics and chemicals to watch for when you shop and select clothing, and how to identify deceptive synthetic fabrics. Labels don't always tell the true story, so you may need to use the series of tests described later, including a safe burn test, to determine whether a fabric is a particular type of synthetic that contains chemicals that you want to avoid.

The Four Stages of Fabric Production

Both synthetic and natural textiles, as they go from fiber to fabric, pass through four distinct production stages. In stage one, fiber preparation, the fibers are cleaned and undergo spinning and weaving. Silk and cotton are usually clean fibers and just require dry processing to remove dirt particles. Raw wool, however, can contain up to 40 percent its weight in impurities that include pesticides, lanolin (wool grease), and dirt and perspiration residues. All require removal and disposal before the next stage of production.

The most common solvent used by manufacturers to clean wool is a chemical called trichloroethylene. This substance has been classified by the International Agency for Research on Cancer as a probable human carcinogen because it induces lung and liver tumors in laboratory test animals. What makes the use of this chemical more distressing is that no safe exposure levels exist, according to the European Union's Existing Chemicals Bureau risk assessment. As the European Union agency reported in 2004: "For carcinogenicity and mutagenicity endpoints there is no identifiable threshold exposure level below which the effects would not be expressed, so there are health concerns at all exposure levels."

In stage two of production, fibers are singed and sized, scoured to further remove impurities, and finally put through a bleaching process that may include optical brightening. During oxidative bleaching, a chemical called EDTA is used, which should be a source of concern for both human health and the environment. This detergent is a proven hormone disrupter, which means it mimics the effects of natural hormones produced by the body's endocrine system. The chemical also persists in effluent released from manufacturing plants, and slow decomposition poses unknown hazards for aquatic and other wildlife.

Concerned by rising EDTA levels measured in its rivers and lakes, Germany forced its textile manufacturers to reduce EDTA releases during the late 1990s and to find safer alternatives that biodegrade rapidly. (In response, German chemists created EDDS and IDA to replace EDTA.)

As for optical brightening, which occurs after bleaching to conceal any discoloration, the chemical agents come from many detergent formulations. Some studies have found that these chemicals also persist in the environment once released in textile effluent. In 2005 the Greenpeace Research Laboratories in Britain did a survey of the scientific literature and found that "there is a general lack of information on toxicity and a need for studies into dermal absorption and the release of these substances from clothes."

Stage three of the production process involves the dyeing or printing of fabrics. Dyes derived from nature pose few health or environmental concerns because natural dyes "tend to be inherently biodegradable and a lower chemical loading to waste streams is associated with their use," according to the Greenpeace report. We are not so fortunate in the case of most synthetic dyes applied to textiles, or in the case of printing pigment processes.

There are a dozen different dye processes and all carry some risks, but the ones with the most problematic health and environmental effects are direct dyes, vat and sulphur dyes, chrome dyes, and most troublesome of all, disperse dyes. Let's look at the problems that Greenpeace identified with each:

- Direct dyes: Saltlike compounds known as quaternary ammonium form with the dye molecules, and the result can be toxic to aquatic organisms. This type of dye is also treated with formaldehyde, whose release with dye waste in effluent creates both ecological and toxicological concerns.
- Vat dyes: These expensive dyes generally involve indigo or anthraquinone colors and may release heavy metals from the production process.
- Sulphur dyes: Sulphide and sodium hydrosulphide are used to make these dyes water soluble, and these can create environmental problems when released into ecosystems.
- Chrome dyes: In this process chrome ions "attach" the fibers to dyestuffs and bonds them to achieve excellent wash fastness. But the use of chromium (VI) can cause allergic skin reactions and even skin ulceration. It can also damage the human kidneys and liver and be toxic to aquatic life. Studies have found that both chromium (III) and chromium (VI) accumulate in many aquatic species, especially in bottom-feeding fish.
- Disperse dyes: These dyes are used to dye polyester. The molecules of this dye are smaller than those of other dyes and "the lack of a strong chemical bond permits a degree of migration out of the fiber (which) accounts for the high incidence of contact dermatitis associated with disperse dye

stuffs," concluded the Greenpeace report. When polyester fabrics treated with these dyes are subjected to high temperatures, antimony oxides are released. These substances are rated by the International Agency for Research on Cancer as a possible carcinogen for humans. At least twenty-one of these dyes have been identified as allergens and the trigger for contact dermatitis.

Dye printing allows textile manufacturers to apply a range of different colors, compared to conventional dyeing that gives fabric a uniform color. But the pigments in printing must be bound to the fabric with a polymer, and the most commonly used plasticizers are a family of phthalates—DEHP, BBP, DINP, and DHP. Phthalates have been well studied and are known to be toxic to both human health and environmental health. DEHP is a reproductive toxin that causes changes in the testes (including atrophy) and damages sperm cells.

Finally, in stage four of textile production, a wide range of finishes are applied depending on the fabric and the claims made by manufacturers to consumers. Some of the claims are ridiculous. For example, there is a "wellness" finish applied by one clothing manufacturer to release the antioxidant vitamin E into the skin of wearers.

Other finishes have received widespread consumer support in the name of convenience—easy care fabrics to bestow wrinkle-resistance and reduce shrinkage from laundering; a variety of waterrepellent finishes; flame retardants in children's clothes and adult's; and antibacterial and fungicidal agents for those concerned with germs. All of these finishes carry some risk to health.

Who knows what else will soon be on the clothing "convenience" horizon (see chapter 7 for some alarming examples.) Today, these are the finishes to watch out for:

- Easy care: Wrinkle-free and shrinkage-free garments release formaldehyde, which is a risk to both human and animal health. Substitutes now exist, if industry will only embrace them, which would eliminate formaldehyde as a by-product of these finishes.
- Waterrepellent: Fluoropolymers are used to repel oil and water from fabric surfaces, but these compounds have proliferated throughout the environment and persist in ecosystems with unknown effects on aquatic and other wildlife.
- Flame retardant: As discussed elsewhere in this book, halogenated flame retardants pose many risks to human and environmental health. Safer alternatives exist, if the textile industry, especially in the United States, just decides to adopt them.
- Bacterial and fungicidal: Triclosan is the most common application in this category of finishes. The Danish EPA has measured triclosan levels in clothes at up to 195 parts per million. It poses health risks for humans and bioaccumulates in

ecosystems, with toxic levels detected in rainbow trout and other aquatic species.

Most recently added to the toxic release load from all of the above is the insecticide called permethrin, which is applied to clothing as an insect killer and has its own documented environmental and health impacts. We will detail those dangers in a later chapter.

You Are Probably Wearing Formaldehyde

Your first and only conscious awareness of contact with formaldehyde may have come in high school biology class when you worked with lab specimens that floated in the preservative, so it may come as a surprise that formaldehyde is also commonly added to clothing to help preserve the fabric from the wear and tear of daily use. You're probably wearing formaldehyde as you read these words.

It was discovered in 1867 by a German scientist who extracted methanol from the charcoaling of wood. A highly toxic chemical, it's effective as a permanent press wrinkle-proofing agent because it's a simple molecule that can connect individual fibers and enable them to hold their shape after repeated cleanings. Other widespread uses of formaldehyde in fabrics, which make it a difficult chemical to avoid, include the following:

- anticling, antistatic, and antishrink finishes to clothing

- waterproof finishes
- perspiration-proof finishes
- moth-proof and mildew-resistant finishes
- stiffening for lightweight nylon knits
- chlorine-resistant finishes
- dyes and printing inks (formaldehyde helps to prevent colors from running by binding the dyes to fabric fibers).

Laboratory testing of animals has documented how formaldehyde acts as a "frank" carcinogen capable of causing cancer in humans. It also can cause a range of other health problems, such as skin and lung irritation, and contact dermatitis. In 2004, the International Agency for Research on Cancer announced that formaldehyde was a probable cause of nasopharyngeal cancer in humans, other evidence linked exposure to nasal cavity and paranasal cavity cancer, while still other studies provided evidence that it might cause leukemia.

When it comes to the presence of formaldehyde in clothing, no country in the world bans its use in textiles, but most governments regulate its levels and some are in disagreement over what levels of this chemical are considered safe for human contact. Here are a few of the limits, based on data compiled in 2008 by the Australian Competition and Consumer Commission:

- In China, the formaldehyde limit is 20ppm (parts per million) in textiles for infants and 75ppm in textiles that will be in direct skin contact with children and adults.

- In Japan, formaldehyde must not be detectable in textiles for infants. For textiles that will be in direct skin contact with children and adults, the limit is 75ppm.
- In the Netherlands, clothing must not contain more than 120ppm after washing.
- In the United States, manufacturers are subject only to "voluntary" standards; no laws or regulations mandate formaldehyde levels.

The attitude of government health and regulatory authorities in the United States toward the presence of formaldehyde in people's lives has provoked considerable concern from independent health and industry experts. David Brookstein, director of the Institute for Textile and Apparel Product Safety, testified in April 2009 before the U.S. Senate Subcommittee on Consumer Protection and made the following declaration about formaldehyde in textiles: "While many industrialized countries limit exposure to formaldehyde in textiles, the United States has only voluntary industry standards. This is a matter of great concern to the American people. The possible health effects from formaldehyde exposure are not fully studied or understood."

What Formaldehyde Levels Are Health Hazards?

Formaldehyde in clothing and its health implications became the focus of a spirited public debate in 2007 when a New Zealand television show broadcast the results of laboratory tests of Chinese clothing imports that apparently found dangerously high levels of the chemical. Concentrations of formaldehyde up to nine hundred times the "safe" level were detected in woolen and cotton clothes manufactured in China, according to TV3's "Target" consumer watchdog program, which had hired an independent laboratory to test children's school clothes, pajamas, trousers, and other garments. The broadcast detailed its findings this way: "The girls' top had a total reading of 230 parts per million, the women's corduroys a total of 290. School shorts total 630. 'Spiderman' T-shirt total 1,400. Pajamas total 3,400, children's pants total 16,000. One hundred percent woolen pants total 17,000, 100 percent cotton trousers total 17,000, and stain-resistant pants total 18,000."

After this controversial program aired, the New Zealand Ministry of Consumer Affairs, under public pressure from clothing importers, did its own testing of formaldehyde in imported fabric and found that "ninety-seven out of the ninety-nine garments it tested had no detectable or very low levels of formaldehyde." This striking discrepancy between the New Zealand TV findings and the government agency results might be explained by a difference in testing procedures and by different points of view about what level of formaldehyde in clothing is really safe.

When the TV show's consulting lab tested the Chinese clothing imports, it measured the combined presence of two types of formaldehyde that appear in fabrics—free and bound. By contrast, the Ministry of Consumer Affairs only measured the clothing for its "free" formaldehyde (molecules unattached to fibers), ignoring the level of bound formaldehyde embedded in the fabric fibers. This is the crux of the reason why some independent health experts dispute the formaldehyde level standards of safety adopted by most governments and the international clothing manufacturing industry, because measuring only the free formaldehyde doesn't tell the complete story of that chemical's presence or effect.

This international standard of measuring clothes only for the free formaldehyde levels present is based on the assumption that bound formaldehyde doesn't off-gas from fabric fibers fast enough, or in great enough quantities, to be absorbed by human skin and pose any hazard to health. So it's never even measured or considered when manufacturers adhere to standards set by the various governments of the world. But is this assumption valid beyond a reasonable doubt, and is it based on solid scientific evidence? The short answer is no!

Consider the implications of how the following study challenges mainstream scientific beliefs. In 1999 a team of Japanese scientists took twenty-seven noniron shirts and measured the quantity of free formaldehyde in each, before and after washing and drying, every week for six months. About one-third of these shirts contained between 75 parts per million and 202ppm of free formaldehyde before washing. After six months, the quantity of free formaldehyde in twelve of the shirts still exceeded 75ppm, which meant that bound formaldehyde in the fabric had continued leaching out over time. A person wearing one of those shirts would have been absorbing a constant stream of formaldehyde molecules for six months. Had the experiment gone on longer, researchers might have found that the exposure extended to a year and beyond. The research team, describing their study results in the *Journal of Health Science,* concluded that "free formaldehyde sometimes increases once again with time by decomposition of (formaldehyde) resin."

There are factors other than just the passage of time involved in the degradation of bound formaldehyde and its release from fabric fibers. Humidity and high temperatures can also cause an increased release of the chemical. Of course, it's precisely the exposure to high heat and humidity that opens up our pores and enables chemicals like formaldehyde to be more readily absorbed. Even the act of sweating, according to the New Zealand Dermatological Society, "appears to leach free formaldehyde from formaldehyde resins" in fabric fibers. Do regulatory agencies take into account all of these factors when deciding what formaldehyde exposure levels in clothing are safe for human health? The short and long answer is no!

The U.S. National Cancer Institute points out that since 1987 the occupational exposure standard for formaldehyde in U.S. workers had been just 1ppm averaged over an eight-hour workday. In 1993, the Occupational Safety and Health Administration changed the law and lowered that standard to only 0.75ppm of exposure. These regulatory changes occurred in the wake of National Cancer Institute findings that a 30 percent increase in lung cancer had developed among workers who were exposed to formaldehyde on the job. Why aren't these same or similar standards of safety being applied to the clothing that people wear eight hours and more a day, every day?

Here is some of what health experts know about the effects of low levels of formaldehyde, especially on children. In the book *Formaldehyde on Trial,* by Lloyd Tataryn, the author observed that "the first adverse health symptoms associated with formaldehyde exposure—burning and tearing of the eyes, general irritation of the upper respiratory tract—usually appear at concentrations beginning at 0.01 parts per million. Concentrations of 0.8 to 1.0ppm can produce bronchitis and asthma. Exposures of 10 to 20ppm can produce severe coughing, a feeling of pressure in the head, headaches, and heart palpitations; exposures of 50 to 100ppm can cause serious lung damage and death."

Dr. Ruth A. Etzel, speaking on behalf of the American Academy of Pediatrics, appeared before the same U.S. Senate Subcommittee in April 2009 that Professor David Brookstein spoke before, and she made these points about formaldehyde in clothing: "Children may be more susceptible than adults to the respiratory effects of formaldehyde. Even at fairly low concentrations, formaldehyde can produce rapid onset of nose and throat irritation, causing cough, chest pain, shortness of breath, and wheezing. At higher levels of exposure, it can cause significant inflammation of the lower respiratory tract, which may result in swelling of the throat, inflammation of the windpipe and bronchi, narrowing of the bronchi, inflammation of the lungs, and accumulation of fluid in the lungs. Children may be more vulnerable than adults to the effects of chemicals like formaldehyde because of the relatively smaller diameter of their airways."

Dr. Etzel strongly urged the U.S. senators, and the Consumer Product Safety Commission, to take action that would "limit formaldehyde in children's clothing." She noted that "at least a dozen other nations already restrict formaldehyde residues in children's clothing," and similar limits should be imposed in the United States. At the very least, she said, the government "should require labels on children's clothing and products that indicate the presence of formaldehyde residues."

Since three-fourths of the clothing sold in the Uunited States each year comes from China and other exporting countries, much of our focus needs to be on whether the formaldehyde standards in those nations are adequate to ensure that manufacturing practices don't endanger health. Professor Andy Pratt with the Department of Chemistry at the University of Canterbury (New Zealand) examined this question and came to some troubling conclusions. "There is a concern that manufacturing processes are not done carefully enough to keep levels of formaldehyde low," he said in an interview. "Formaldehyde levels are much higher than we've seen in the past. We've seen this through the increasing production of fabrics in Eastern Europe and in China. The traditional safety levels in many of those clothing manufacturing plants have not been at the level we've expected in western countries, and as you drop those standards of tract chemical contamination, you end up with this problem."

The following points summarize the case against the use of formaldehyde in clothing and why you should avoid any garments containing this chemical:

- Both free and bound levels of formaldehyde in garments should be measured together and taken into account to establish standards of health and safety, because the bound levels migrate out of fabric fibers and into skin contact much more easily and frequently than clothing manufacturers or regulatory agencies seem aware or will publicly acknowledge.

- Clothing imported from China and other newly industrialized countries contains higher levels of formaldehyde than previously allowed, and this clothing now accounts for most of the wearing apparel sold in the United States and many other western countries. (An investigation by the Australian Wool Testing Authority that was reported by *The Sydney Morning Herald* in 2007, for example, found that a brand of blanket imported from China contained 2,790 parts per million of formaldehyde, more than ten times the amount permissible under any international standard.)
- It's not just the levels of formaldehyde that our skin is exposed to in clothing that we should be concerned about. We also absorb formaldehyde from multiple sources every day, such as cosmetics and other personal care products that we also put on our skin. We must think in terms of reducing our exposure levels from *all* of these many sources of contamination.
- Finally, though clothing manufacturers contend that low levels of formaldehyde exposure from their garments will have no health effects, these reassurances fail to take into account the cumulative long-term effect in the human body from absorbing formaldehyde molecules as clothing degrades with washing.

Even Cotton Conceals Chemical Dangers

Most consumers assume that if an item of clothing is labeled as "cotton" or even "natural," it must automatically be a safe product. But it's important to keep in mind that not all cotton is created equal. Non-organic cotton contains residues of herbicides and pesticides that are used in the growing process. These can be detrimental to human health, especially infant and child health.

There are many reasons for choosing organic cotton over nonorganic cotton varieties, and not just for human health reasons. We lessen our impact on the environment by choosing organic brands of clothing.

What does organic really mean when applied to cotton garments? As defined by the National Organic Standards board, "Organic agriculture is an ecological production management system that promotes and enhances biodiversity, biological cycles, and soil biological activity. It is based on the minimal use of off-farm inputs and on management practices that restore, maintain, and enhance ecological harmony." In other words, organic means the use of few if any synthetic chemicals in the cultivation of cotton, or in the manufacturing process.

Because cotton isn't a food crop, the herbicides and pesticides and other chemicals used in the production of nonorganic varieties aren't regulated by the government. Cotton is the most pesticide-dependent crop grown anywhere in the world, accounting for 25 percent of all pesticide use. So for every single pair of jeans and every T-shirt produced using cotton, about one pound of pesticides and chemical fertilizers are used.

During the conversion of conventional cotton into clothing, still more toxic chemicals are added at each stage of its production, from harsh petroleum scours, softeners, brighteners, and heavy metals to flame and soil retardants, ammonia, and formaldehyde, and finally, synthetic chemical dyes. Many of these toxins have been linked to a range of health problems, including allergies, insomnia, immune disorders, cancer, and neurological disorders.

A virtual witch's brew of toxins are absorbed by the cotton fibers by the time it reaches consumers. Because a baby's skin is more porous, thinner, and more absorbent than an adult's, we must be particularly vigilant about their skin contact with nonorganic cotton. The manufacturer Johnson & Johnson makes the following point on the company website: "A baby's skin is thinner, more fragile, and less oily than an adult's. A baby's skin also produces less melanin, the substance that helps protect against sunburn. It's less resistant to bacteria and harmful substances in the environment, especially if it's irritated. Babies also sweat less efficiently than the rest of us, so it's harder for them to maintain their inner body temperature."

Organic clothing uses cotton that is farmed without pesticides and involves safer methods, such as crop rotation, physical removal of weeds instead of use of herbicides, hand hoeing, and the introduction of beneficial insects such as ladybugs to counteract the presence of pests. The result is a cotton fabric that is toxin free and kid friendly.

Producers of organic cotton claim a variety of other benefits from its use—it's safer, sturdier, cheaper, and feels better on the skin. Conventionally produced cotton material may only last for ten to twenty washes before it starts to break down, whereas organic cotton fabric can last for one hundred washes or more before it begins to show wear. The reason for this difference is that conventionally produced cotton fibers take so much abuse—going through scouring, bleaching, dying, softeners, formaldehyde spray, and flame and soil retardants—before even being shipped to be cut for patterns that result in the clothing you see in stores.

Choosing organic fibers is another step toward more natural and more healthful living. To summarize, here are our top seven reasons to tell yourself and others that organic cotton is superior to nonorganic blends:

1. It helps to protect your and your children's health.
2. It reduces pesticide and other chemical use.
3. It protects farm workers from chemical exposure.
4. It helps to protect water and overall environmental quality.

5. It is a sturdier and longer-lasting fabric.
6. It feels more comfortable to wear.
7. It supports a more sustainable future for agriculture.

How Much Flame Retardant Have You Absorbed?

It seemed like a good idea at the time—make children's sleepwear self-extinguishing if the clothing caught on fire. What could possibly be wrongheaded about such a worthy goal of protecting our children?

After the U.S. Consumer Product Safety Commission (CPSC) ruled in 1971 that children's sleepwear must be self-extinguishing when exposed to heat or flames, clothing manufacturers began adding a fire retardant chemical called brominated Tris to children's clothing fabrics. Amounts equal to about 5 percent of the fabric weight were added to each piece of sleepwear to make it flame resistant.

Odds are that if you or your child were born or grew up during the 1970s, you were exposed to Tris. Fibers used in children's sleepwear that were treated with it included acetate, triacetate, and polyester. The CPSC estimated that 120 million sleepwear garments contained this flame retardant, and we can assume, based on cultural practices of that time, that many of those garments were passed down within families to each newborn child until the clothing wore out, which means human skin was in contact with the retardant chemical well into the 1980s.

Chemists Arlene Blum and Bruce Ames at the University of California, Berkeley, tested the brominated Tris flame retardant and discovered that it was a human carcinogen (cancer causing) and published their findings in a 1977 issue of the journal *Science.* Subsequently, Blum and Ames did a second study, also published in *Science,* which revealed an equally alarming discovery—children were absorbing the flame retardant.

Morning urine samples were taken from ten children who wore either pajamas newly treated with Tris or older pajamas treated with Tris but washed numerous times. Most of the pajamas were made of polyester. Tris residue was found in the urine of every child, and it had to have come from absorbing the chemical by contact with the pajamas because Tris isn't normally found in nature or in human bodies.

The idea that repeated washings of the clothes would remove the Tris and pose less of a health hazard to wearers was directly contradicted by this study. A separate experiment was cited in which the total Tris in a fabric only decreased from 5.8 percent to 5.1 percent of weight after *more than fifty washings* of the fabric. "Tris is likely to continue diffusing from the inside of the fiber to the outside as the garment is being worn, leading to continuing availability of the chemical for absorption through the skin or by mouth," concluded Blum and Ames. "Repeatedly washed Tris sleepwear still contains large amounts of the chemical and is likely to pose a continuing hazard."

Here is how the two chemists described the "grave threat to human health" that Tris posed to children: brominated Tris is a mutagen and causes cancer and sterility in animals. Mutagen means that it can cause inheritable mutations in humans, damaging the DNA. They wrote: "Potential adverse reproductive effects from brominated Tris are also a concern. This chemical causes testicular atrophy and sterility." Of particular concern for male children, Tris can be absorbed through the scrotum because it's "about twenty times more permeable to chemicals than is other skin."

Based on the Blum and Ames findings, along with separate National Cancer Institute research that shows Tris to cause cancer in laboratory test animals, an organization called the Environmental Defense Fund filed a petition with the CPSC seeking the chemical's removal from children's clothing. The CPSC acted by issuing a ban on the sale of any more children's sleepwear containing this chemical, but the agency *did not* recall from public circulation the already-sold garments containing this toxic chemical.

This toxin came into contact with the skin of an estimated fifty million children in the United States and even after its dangers were exposed, the federal regulatory agency allowed these contaminated garments to stay in public use, being absorbed by still more children, for many more years to come. But believe it or not, this isn't the only Tris-related affront to human health that occurred!

Once the clothing industry abandoned the brominated Tris retardant, companies replaced it with dichlorinated Tris, which proved to be nearly as toxic. Another study published in *Science* by Blum and Ames, this time in 1978, showed that the new type of Tris retardant was a hazard to human health in many of the same ways that its cousin had been documented to be. This science paper also resulted in the CPSC taking action, but this time it was with a polite rebuke that merely requested that clothing manufacturers not use this second type of Tris in clothing any more.

Trade Secrecy Law Conceals Health Threats

Today, most synthetic fabrics for children's sleepwear contain a new generation of flame retardants that are bonded into the fabric. These retardants must survive at least fifty washings of the clothing. But as for the identity of the chemicals being used to meet flammability standards, nonindustry chemists can only make educated guesses.

After the twin Tris debacles, chemical companies began hiding the identity of the flame retardant chemicals being used in clothing by taking advantage of U.S. laws that are designed to protect patents from infringement by competitors. Chemical mixtures that met CPSC flammability standards for fabrics became "proprietary" information in the United States, with many clothing manufacturers even being denied access to the identities of chemicals in flame retardants they were purchasing from chemical companies. As Professor Blum told us: "Today, you can't find out what's in most formulations. They're not required to reveal chemical identities or health data about their use."

Science magazine Editor-in-Chief Donald Kennedy editorialized about this problem for consumers in a November 2007 issue: "The laws and rules regarding the introduction of toxic chemicals into consumer products and the environment are still ineffectual. The U.S. regulatory system for toxic industrial chemicals is not effective and is a threat to public health." Kennedy called for the U.S. Congress to enact "a real proof-of-safety provision" for fire retardants and other chemicals to "stop the chemical industry from continuing to make consumer protection look like a game of whack-a-mole."

Independent chemists in the United States and Europe who we consulted for this book did speculate about which flame-retardant chemicals are now being used in U.S.-sold clothing in order to meet CPSC flammability regulations. Usually these are retardants banned by the European Union as potential health hazards under the Registration, Evaluation, and Authorization of Chemicals (REACH) standards that Europe began implementing at the turn of this century.

A chemist in Sweden informed us that "a fair guess is that halogenated triaryl phosphonates are used for children's clothing and sleepwear, due to their low negative influence on the good comfort and durability properties of the fabric. Some of these flame retardants are reproductive toxic." In other words, any parent concerned about his or her child's health over the course of a lifetime should never purchase clothing containing those chemicals. Halogenated chemicals can bioaccumulate (collect in body tissues) and have been documented as being capable of causing cancer and endocrine system disorders in lab animals.

A family of fire-retardant chemicals called PBDEs are also a major cause of health concern. There are three types: penta, used in furniture foam; octa, used in hard electrical plastic; and deca, found in some textiles. These chemicals delay ignition of products exposed to flames but don't stop fires, and at low temperature combustion, they release high levels of brominated dioxins, which are toxic substances. In 2004, manufacturers of penta voluntarily ceased production because of serious health and environmental repercussions that could have subjected the companies to costly lawsuits. Whereas octa has been shown in lab tests on animals to induce fetal toxicity, and some studies show deca to be a carcinogen at high levels of exposure and a toxin to thyroid, liver, and kidney function, yet both of these types of PBDE's remain in wide use.

A review of all published scientific studies on the toxic effects of PBDEs on humans and wildlife, conducted in 2003 by a scientist with the Swedish National Food Administration, found three categories of health concerns from PBDE exposure: neurobehavioral development; thyroid hormone levels; and at higher levels of exposure, PB-DEs can be carcinogenic. Studies done by the Environmental Working Group in the United States tested the blood of entire families and detected these fire retardants in toddlers and preschoolers at levels *three times higher* than in their mother's bodies. Previous testing had found PBDEs appearing in the breast milk of most nursing mothers who have been tested. These retardant chemicals are bioaccumulating in both humans and wildlife because they persist in the environment, and once absorbed by living flesh, persist in body tissues.

You might also be interested (and alarmed) to know that the same type of Tris (chlorinated) that was removed from children's pajamas as a health hazard in 1977 is now being used in your upholstered furniture foam, as well as in baby carriers and bassinets. "The same chlorinated Tris is currently the second most used fire retardant in foam in furniture in the United States," points out Dr. Arlene Blum, "used in levels up to 5 percent of the weight of the foam. Tris is a mutagen and a carcinogen." She appeared before the CPSC in November 2007 and urged the agency to take these three steps to protect public health:

1. All flame-retardant chemicals should be required to be shown safe for human health and the environment before the chemicals are allowed to be used in products.
2. More research and development resources should be devoted to developing nontoxic, "green" flame retardants.
3. A moratorium should be imposed on new flammability regulations until new "green" flame retardants are developed, or existing flame retardants are demonstrated to be safe.

"We continue to move from one toxic fire retardant chemical to another," declared Dr. Blum. "Toxic PBDEs were used to treat furniture foam from the early 1980s until they were banned by the California legislature and the manufacturer ceased production in 2004. They were replaced by chlorinated Tris, a known toxicant, and also unknown proprietary mixtures containing chemical cousins."

How much of a problem do fire hazards really pose to children's clothing? Can flame retardants in sleepwear even be justified any more?

The answer, as provided by the U.S. Consumer Product Safety Commission's National Burn Center Reporting System, may surprise you. Each year, on average, only about thirty-six cases of serious injury from children's sleepwear catching fire are reported throughout the United States. Since these thirty-six cases usually involve sleepwear treated with fire retardants, the question becomes one of public health: is the risk of contaminating millions of children with toxic fire retardants and endangering their health worth protecting the thirty-six children each year who benefit from wearing the chemical?

Ultimately, only parents acting on their own can answer those questions and make that decision by voting with their pocketbooks. Only they can accept or reject clothing that is questionable for their children's health.

Most Common Chemicals in Clothes

You are shopping for a new dress or a new suit, and you want a stain-resistant and wrinkle-resistant fabric. What are you really putting on your skin when you buy such a product? What health considerations are you sacrificing in the name of convenience? Formaldehyde, a frank carcinogen shown in lab testing of animals to cause cancer, is but one of the toxic chemicals used in these fabrics. As stated earlier, most clothing is now manufactured in China, where permissible levels of formaldehyde are higher than EPA standards for U.S manufacturers.

Children are particularly vulnerable to chemical sensitivities triggered by the clothing they wear, especially if they are required to wear uniforms during the school year. Many school uniforms are coated with a family of chemicals called PFCs that give fabrics stain resistance and the "noniron" wrinkle resistance often found in school trousers and skirts. These perfluorinated compounds have been classified as probable cancer-causative agents by the EPA.

As clothes containing these chemicals become worn with repeated washings and wear, the chemicals migrate from the fabric and become particles that can be absorbed or inhaled by children. "Without knowing it, parents are exposing their children to toxic chemicals in clothing that could have serious future consequences for their health and the environment," declared Dr. Richard Dixon, head of the environmental group WWF Scotland, in a 2004 media alert. "Children are usually more vulnerable to the effects of chemicals than adults, so the presence of these substances in school clothing is particularly alarming."

Studies done by the Environmental Working Group in the United States have detected PFOA, one of the common Teflon-like chemicals, in the blood of 96 percent of all Americans tested. In 2004 another study by the same organization examined umbilical cord blood donated by U.S. hospitals, and found eight types of perfluorochemicals in nearly all of the samples, demonstrating that mothers absorb the chemicals during everyday activities and then transfer the toxins directly to the fetuses they carry.

Buy Nontoxic Children's Sleepwear

You don't need to subject your child to playing the role of guinea pig in any flame retardant sleepwear experiments in which the child's long-term health is placed in jeopardy by chemicals without proven records of safety.

In 1996 the Consumer Product Safety Commission created an exemption to its flammability standards for children's sleepwear. Any garments for infants nine months of age or younger, and tight-fitting sleepwear for children older than nine months, were excluded from the requirement of being manufactured with flame-retardant chemicals bonded into the fabric. The requirement for flame retardants remains in effect for all other types of clothing sleepwear.

Labels that say "wear snug fitting" must be attached to any sleepwear that doesn't contain flame retardants, which is a requirement that went into effect on June 28, 2000, for all cotton or cotton blend snug-fitting clothing used by children. Loose-fitting T-shirts and other loose-fitting clothing made of cotton or cotton blends, according to the CPSC, shouldn't be used for sleeping because "these garments can catch fire easily, burn rapidly, and are associated with nearly three hundred emergency-room-treated burn injuries to children each year."

What exactly is considered children's sleepwear by the CPSC? The agency identifies the garments as any article of clothing, such as pajamas, a nightgown, a robe, or loungewear, that is sized for kids above nine months of age and up to size 14; the garment must be worn primarily for sleeping. Diapers and underwear aren't considered sleepwear according to this definition.

Numerous clothing companies now sell CPSC-approved pajamas and other sleepwear without flame retardants. Two of the more prominent manufacturers are L.L. Bean (www.llbean.com) and Lands' End (www.landsend.com).

The long-term health consequences of this contamination in the unborn remain in the realm of speculation for two reasons: (1) these contaminants are now so prevalent in humans and wildlife that they can't be separated from the presence of other toxic chemicals that are being absorbed simultaneously; and (2) these chemicals were only introduced into clothing and other consumer products within the past few decades, so we don't have evidence generated by a lifetime of use. But we feel assured that PFCs that are absorbed from clothing and other sources can't be safe for children or the rest of us.

CHAPTER 3

Health Effects of Synthetics

Our Toxic Chemical "Body Burden"

Each and every one of us carries around a "body burden" of synthetic chemicals that we have absorbed from our foods, medicines, and consumer products. These chemicals, once taken in through our skin or lungs or by digestion, take up residence in our body fat and our body organs. Over time, as the toxins from multiple sources accumulate, we begin to experience the health consequences in the form of a weakened immune system and resultant illness and disease.

Since 2001 blood studies done by the U.S. Centers for Disease Control and Prevention (CDC), involving more than ten thousand people of all ages and backgrounds, found that every American carries a body burden of at least seven hundred or more synthetic chemicals. These are conservative estimates because the CDC has tested humans for only a few thousand of the more than 85,000 chemicals now in commercial use in the United States.

What all of us, not just prospective mothers, should find even more disturbing is the extent to which this body burden of chemicals is being passed on to future generations while they are still in the womb. In a 2004 study by the Environmental Working Group (EWG), two testing laboratories measured the chemical toxins in umbilical cord blood taken from U.S. hospitals. On average about two hundred synthetic chemicals were detected in the umbilical cord samples. Both flame retardants and pesticides were among the chemical residues found, as well as the Teflon chemical called PFOA, all of which may appear on, or in, new clothing. Most of the toxins that were discovered have been shown in medical studies to be possible or probable causes of birth defects, developmental disorders, nervous system disorders, and cancer.

Chemical contamination from clothing alone, of course, doesn't account for this body burden of toxins. Much of the burden comes from the chemical ingredients in cosmetics and personal care products simply because those chemicals are applied directly to the skin on a daily basis. But chemicals from synthetic clothing do contribute to the body burden and may even be one of the "tipping points" for triggering immune system collapse and the onset of illness and disease.

Manufacturers of consumer products try to reassure us that the tiny levels of chemicals in their products don't do any harm to our health in either the short term or the long term. Even if that were true, it's a rationale that ignores several discomfiting facts that mainstream toxicologists are finally beginning to acknowledge and take into account.

One is the health impact of bioaccumulation within the human body. We know that many toxins persist in our bodies and in the environment. Many of these chemicals were designed to be virtually immortal and don't break down easily. Once in human body fat, these chemicals accumulate over a lifetime with a variety of potential effects on health.

A second and even more unpredictable reality is that many of these synthetic chemicals combine with each other to create synergies. These are processes in which the health effect of two or more chemicals acting together is much more powerful than any one of the chemicals can have on its own. This is mostly uncharted research territory for medical science, toxicologists, and product manufacturers simply because the costs are too prohibitive to create the technology necessary to do the wide range of testing that takes into account the billions of different chemical synergy combinations.

It's a mind-boggling task to try and predict which synergies are occurring within us. We can only fall back on two proven ways to protect ourselves: first, limit our exposure to synthetic chemicals in whatever ways we can, which means buying and wearing only natural organic clothing, along with using organic foods and personal care products; and second, periodically undertake detoxification regimens to leach accumulated chemicals out of our body fat and organs.

Chemical Sensitivity Is Spreading

Back in the 1950s an allergist practicing in the United States, Dr. Theron Randolph, began to notice that some of his patients seemed to have physical reactions to many of the new conveniences of modern life. They were becoming ill from contact with chemicals in consumer products that manufacturers and mainstream toxicologists considered safe in their exposure levels.

Upon further investigation, Dr. Randolph concluded that his patients simply couldn't adapt to these newly formulated chemicals. The analogy he thought of to account for this inability to adapt likened the human immune system to a barrel. As the body continually absorbs chemicals, eventually the "barrel" overflows, and physical symptoms appear as a reaction to the chemical overload. The toxins have accumulated until they overwhelmed the body's mechanisms for eliminating them.

Multiple Chemical Sensitivities became the medical term to describe the syndrome of symptoms that began to afflict some people. Reported symptoms include headaches, loss of concentration, itching, tingling sensations, hives, dizziness, nausea, irritability, insomnia, nervousness, and depression.

In clothing, the chemicals and fabrics that can trigger this syndrome range from formaldehyde to polyester, and from pesticide residues to the polyethylene plastics that constitute fake leather.

Some people can detoxify these chemicals faster and easier than other people. But ultimately, we are all at risk, no matter how healthy our body's detoxification system may be, because we are constantly being bombarded by new chemicals and intensifying levels of chemicals.

Over the past decade, considerable medical research has demonstrated how the barrel analogy works in principle in humans and other forms of life. For instance, a 2001 study in the journal *Brain Research* showed how repeated low-level exposures to formaldehyde made test animals much more reactive to future exposure to formaldehyde.

"People concerned about chemical overloads," says Michael Lackman of Lotus Organics, "should be 'anti' any garment that is advertised as being antishrink, antibacterial, antimicrobial, antistatic, antiodor, antiflame, antiwrinkle, antistain, or any of the other 'anti' easy care garment finishes."

Every product sold on the market that touches our skin is a test of our sensitivity because the chemical ingredients in the product are usually untested for their impact on human health before marketing occurs, which makes us all guinea pigs in an uncontrolled experiment. When these experiments go awry, it is sometimes the most vulnerable among us—infants—who become the first health statistics.

A textbook example of our guinea pig status occurred in 2008, when graphic reports surfaced about a particular product line of baby clothes. John Kunze of San Francisco told a reporter for NBC Los Angeles that a rash had appeared on his daughter's back while she was wearing Carter's tagless baby clothes: "It (the rash) was bright red. It was oozing, weeping. It was just bad." His daughter, Ava, suffered for months, was admitted on two occasions to emergency rooms, and accumulated $10,000 in medical bills.

"I can't tell you how frustrated I was," said her mother, Janet Kunze. "This could have all been avoided had they (Carter's) disclosed at least a warning that these were hazardous clothes."

Other parents who had purchased the same clothing described how their infants developed serious rashes that resembled burns, and in some cases, patches of the children's skin came off when their pajamas were removed. Pediatricians who examined the children said the injuries looked like chemical burns. Hundreds more parents came forward with their own horror stories in postings on the Internet. Here are just a few of the heartrending and angry comments that parents posted on a media website in November 2008:

- Jeni wrote, "Our pediatrician said the rash on my daughter would go away, but it doesn't. It just gets bigger, oozes, and then flakes off like a burn or a welt. I cannot imagine the scar it will leave on her!"
- Greg wrote, "My son has been having this same issue. He has suffered for almost two years now. He has mild to severe rashes, weeping, itching,

and unbelievably disturbing to look at. He has seen his pediatrician and three specialists numerous times, and the doctors had no diagnoses."

- Christina wrote, "For months my daughter has been scratching her neck, the back of her head, and behind her ears, until she bleeds! I've changed the soap, shampoo, lotion, and her diet, thinking one of these things might be the cause. I can't believe it's the clothing I've been putting her in. Makes total sense and makes me feel awful!"

In response to this upsurge of complaints, the U.S. Consumer Product Safety Commission eventually issued an advisory that warned parents that the Carter's fall 2007 product line of clothing for infants and children could cause allergic reactions—contact dermatitis—possibly due to chemicals in labels on the inside back of the garments. The clothing had been made in China and several other countries, but the labels were manufactured in the United States. Despite this advisory, Carter's Inc. of Atlanta, Georgia, didn't seek a recall of the hazardous garments. Though most of the medical conditions were caused by the Carter's products, several other brands of infant clothing, among them Baby Gap and Circo, were also singled out by parents as causing allergic reactions.

Contact dermatitis is a group of skin conditions, including eczema, that affects both children and adults. In the 1960s, only about 3 percent of children had the condition according to public health agencies, but by the year 2000, an estimated 20 percent of all children suffered from it at some point in their development. Why the sharp increase in just a generation? It probably wasn't a coincidence that the skin problems multiplied and intensified during the same period of time that synthetic clothing dominated sales in the industrialized countries of the world. Nor should it be a surprise that most manufacturers refuse to accept any real responsibility for the effect their chemical clothing is having on human health.

In the case of Carter's sleepwear, the company did send refunds to any parents who requested them (an estimated one thousand consumers made contact with the company over this issue) but otherwise, company officials refused to pay medical bills for injured children, or even to acknowledge that any chemical in their clothing could be to blame for the allergic reactions. The company's position was explained on its website this way: "We have conducted an internal review of the product and test results, required of our label manufacturers to do the same, and coordinated with several independent experts, including physicians, to provide their analyses. Our review and testing provide no indication that the labels contain any known skin irritants or abrasive chemicals, or that such a rash is anything beyond a rare allergic reaction to an otherwise safe product."

Though the labels Carter's used reportedly contained the same standard ink formulations employed by many companies, some observers detected evidence that the allergic reactions may have resulted from the company making a switch from natural fabric labels to synthetic labels. "The exact chemical formulations and ingredients of such products are carefully guarded trade secrets," wrote a commentator on the Z Recommends website, which is devoted to safer children's products, "and may not even be available to the companies that make use of them."

Carter's Inc. CEO Michael Casey did an interview with Z Recommends and in it claimed that "there was nothing in that label we could identify that could cause that kind of reaction which led us to conclude that this is a rare allergic reaction in some babies with highly sensitive skin." Numerous readers of the website responded to this claim by echoing an observation made by a mother named Jenna: "A niggling little thing about what I keep reading that irks me is that they keep referring to this as being a problem for babies with 'very sensitive skin.' My daughter has never had sensitive skin. She never had any other skin rash. She doesn't even get diaper rash. So it bugs me a little that they seem to want to fob off this problem as a fault of my child's skin rather than a fault of their product."

Why Contact Dermatitis Is More Common

As synthetic clothing dyes and garment finishes became more common and widespread on store shelves, so did the variety of reported health problems and chemical sensitivities experienced by ever-greater numbers of people of all ages. Skin rashes, nausea, fatigue, burning, itching, headaches, difficulty breathing—these are just a few of the symptoms associated with chemical clothing sensitivity. Children have their own additional list of symptoms that includes flushed cheeks, hyperactivity, and even learning and behavioral problems.

Garment finishes that are applied to new clothing constitute a long list and can usually be identified by their function. If your clothing is described as flame retardant or resistant, stain resistant, wrinkle free, antistatic, odor resistant, permanent press, nonshrink, antifungal, or antibacterial, you can be pretty sure that synthetic chemicals were either directly applied to the fabric or bonded into the fabric, and the residue can induce allergic reactions in some people.

Avoid These Textile Dye Allergens and Carcinogens

Synthetic dyes used in clothing are the primary culprits in the spread of allergic dermatitis among a large percentage of the industrialized world's population. Some dyes are also carcinogens (cancer-causing agents.) Here are the worst allergen and carcinogen offenders that have been identified in dye dermatitis studies over the past two decades. Results were published in the *Journal of the American Academy of Dermatology,* the *American Journal of Contact Dermatology,* and other peer-reviewed medical science journals. In addition, here is a list of dye carcinogens compiled by the Norwegian Textile Panel and chemists in Sweden.

Allergens

Disperse Blue 3
Disperse Blue 7
Disperse Blue 24
Disperse Blue 26
Disperse Blue 35
Disperse Blue 85
Disperse Blue 102
Disperse Blue 106
Disperse Blue 124
Disperse Blue 153
Disperse Red 1
Disperse Red 11

Disperse Red 17
Disperse Yellow 1
Disperse Yellow 3
Disperse Yellow 9
Disperse Yellow 39
Disperse Yellow 49
Disperse Orange 1
Disperse Orange 3
Disperse Orange 13
Basic Black 1
Basic Brown 1
Disperse Brown 1
Basic Red 46
Supramine Yellow
Supramine Red
Diazol Orange
Neutrichrome Red

Carcinogens

Acid Red 26
Basic Red 9
Basic Violet 14
Direct Black 38
Direct Blue 6
Direct Brown 95
Direct Red 28
Disperse Blue 1
Disperse Orange 11
Disperse Orange 149

Clothing dyes present an even more complex challenge to human health. It's not just the vast array of chemical dye colors that can trigger reactions, it's the chemicals used in the dyeing process that sometimes linger, hidden in clothing fabrics and absorbed by the skin. Some of the toxins used to bond dye colors to fabric include formaldehyde (a known carcinogen), dioxin (a carcinogen and hormone disrupter), and metals like chrome and copper.

Consider for a moment formaldehyde's role in causing contact dermatitis, which has been the subject of numerous medical science studies and journal articles. Uniforms of all types have been identified as primary culprits in releasing formaldehyde into human skin and the surrounding environment.

A 2007 article in the medical journal *Dermatitis* described how a 49-year-old pediatrician developed "a severe widespread dermatitis caused by contact with formaldehyde textile resins from her hospital 'greens' (scrubs) and mask." The two authors of this study commented that "despite a trend for reduction in the concentration of free formaldehyde in textiles, formaldehyde textile resin allergic contact dermatitis remains an important clinical issue and is likely underdiagnosed." Not only that, but diagnosis is made more problematic because "patch testing with the suspected offending fabric often leads to false-negative results."

Other studies have found excessive formaldehyde in uniforms worn by military personnel and airline employees. Formaldehyde's appearance in permanent press clothing, in both uniforms and everyday wear, and the resulting cases of contact dermatitis "is more common than has been previously recognized," reported a 1992 study published in the *Journal of the American Academy of Dermatology.* That shouldn't be surprising since formaldehyde resins have been used to impart wrinkle resistance to fabrics since the late 1920s. What should surprise and concern anyone, however, is that formaldehyde continues to be used even though it has been shown to cause cancer in laboratory testing of animals.

Many Consumers Are Sensitive to Disperse Blue Dyes

Synthetic garments colored in shades of Disperse Blue may look gorgeous and even regal, yet with this family of dyes, looks really can be dangerously deceiving. Of all the synthetic dyes that cause allergic dermatitis—and there are dozens—the Disperse Blue family ranks as the ruler over them all.

Proof of their status came in 2004 at the end of an exhaustive four-year study of 644 people in Israel who were suspected to have contact dermatitis stemming from textiles they wore. Headed by Dr. Aneta Lazarov, who is affiliated with the Sackler School of Medicine at Tel Aviv University, the study patch tested 441 women and 203 men multiple times. She presented the results at the 12th Congress of the European Academy of Dermatology and Venereology.

The clothing most likely to trigger contact dermatitis contained synthetic dyes that were dark blue, brown, and black, which are also the ones most likely to contain Disperse Blue dyes. The problem clothes were all synthetic. Silk and pure cotton garments seldom caused a reaction.

Nearly 31 percent of the positive dye reactions occurred with Disperse Blue 124, about 27 percent with Disperse Blue 106, and nearly 10 percent with Disperse Blue 85. Numerous patients were allergic to multiple types of Disperse Blue dyes. Some patients developed serious lesions in locations on their body where synthetic clothing rubbed or was snug, such as the waist and inner thighs. Forty of the test subjects also had a reaction to formaldehyde and textile finish resins that remained in fabrics.

"Once patients have become sensitized to a dye and/or resin in synthetic clothing, usually the problem won't disappear with laundering," Dr. Lazarov observed. This is important for consumers to keep in mind when purchasing clothes. Even miniscule levels of a chemical toxin in a fabric—no matter how many times it's washed—can continue to trigger health problems for someone with a chemical sensitivity.

At least one Disperse Blue dye can cause health problems that are much more serious than contact dermatitis. In the *Report on Carcinogens, Eleventh Edition,* published by the National Institutes of Health, animal studies done on Disperse Blue 1 were evaluated and the conclusion was reached that the dye "is reasonably anticipated to be a human carcinogen based on evidence of malignant tumor formation in experimental animals to an unusual degree."

This report identified Disperse Blue 1 as "a fabric dye for nylon, cellulose acetate and triacetate, polyester, and acrylate fibers ... and also used to dye fur, sheepskin, acetate, nylon, and other synthetic fibers." Like so many other chemicals used in synthetic clothing, this dye appears in cosmetics and personal care products, particularly in semipermanent formulations of hair dyes.

Despite the evidence for this dye's cancer-causing potential, the dye's use and sale continues without meaningful restrictions or warnings. In fact, for all of the 1990s "the total production volume of all Disperse Blue dyes was unreported," meaning that no one knows how many people might have been exposed to it. As the *Report on Carcinogens* commented, "No specific regulations or guidelines relevant to reduction of exposure to Disperse Blue 1 were identified."

Cancer-Causing Dyes in Chinese-Made Clothing

An alarming sixty-five separate clothing brands in China were found to contain toxic dyes that are known cancer-causing agents, or they failed to meet other basic quality standards, according to a 2010 investigation by Beijing's Bureau of Industry and Commerce. Many clothes produced by these brands were exported to the United States and other Western countries.

Some of the clothing brands contained excessive levels of formaldehyde, a well-known carcinogen that can be absorbed by human skin. Others contained decomposable aromatic amines, a cancer-causing textile dye that is also easily absorbed by human skin.

It may sound absurd to believe that a T-shirt or a pair of pants could cause cancer, but the threat certainly exists when repeated use places the wearer's skin in constant contact with known toxic chemicals. Though the garments were withdrawn from the marketplace in China after these revelations, those already shipped overseas are still being worn by unsuspecting consumers.

Synthetic Fibers Fatigue Your Muscles

Medical studies have shown that there is a huge difference in the ways that natural fibers and synthetic fibers affect muscle performance. This will come as news to high-performance athletes, for whom it could make the difference between winning and losing, and it will surprise ordinary consumers who wear synthetics and wonder why they feel fatigued every day.

In an eye-opening study from 2001 that got little or no attention in the United States, five physiologists from Poland compared muscle function in the forearms of test subjects who wore either natural or synthetic fiber clothing. They published their findings in the journal *Fibres & Textiles in Eastern Europe.* This may not seem like a significant issue to study at first blush. After all, you may wonder what possible difference lightweight fabrics can make in your muscle strength and endurance. It turns out that the difference in the effects between natural and synthetic fibers can influence performance for a wide variety of professionals—from people who sit at computers for long hours to manual laborers to professional athletes.

Twelve male volunteers, aged twenty-four to twenty-seven, all of whom were in good health, wore long-sleeve shirts made of linen for about five hours, and then wore similar shirts made of polyester for another five hours. Their forearm muscles were monitored with electrodes that measured skin temperature and the conduction velocity of motor fibers in the muscle. This was done as they worked at computers, read books, or just conversed with each other.

No negative changes in muscle functioning were observed when the test subjects wore the natural linen fabric shirts. However, a range of muscle disruptions occurred when the men wore the polyester shirts. The first major difference was that the synthetic fabric created an electrostatic field emission over the surface of the muscle, which the natural fabric didn't create. A second major effect was that "covering the surface of the forearm caused the temperature to increase significantly in the subjects dressed in the synthetic clothing." Conduction velocities in the motor fibers within the nerve branches of the muscle underwent a lower amplitude when the test subjects wore the synthetic shirts.

Here is how the study authors summarized their findings: "Temporarily covering the tested forearm muscles with synthetic clothing changes the pattern of motor unit activity. This is expressed by the low-frequency spontaneous activity of the muscle fibers during the state of rest, or by diminished high-frequency activity of the muscle units during the voluntary movements ... fluctuations are the reason for the desynchronization in muscle motor units that may lead to a greater tendency to fatigue while wearing the synthetic garments ... the electric charges gathered on the polyester cloth surface which cause an electrostatic field on the skin-cloth zone, together with an increase in the skin temperature in the polyester cloth, may be the cause for the observed changes."

Still another finding and observation from this study may prove useful for those of you who must choose between natural or synthetic fabrics during cold weather: "The higher level of heat resistance of linen cloth demonstrates its better thermal protection against cold than in the case with polyester cloth."

Synthetics Can Warp Male Sexuality

Though he had never been known as a "high-energy" kind of guy, fifty-eight-year-old office cleaner Frank Clewer certainly made the sparks fly one day in September 2005 when he was job hunting in Warrnambool, a town in western Australia. Wearing several items of synthetic clothing, including a zip-up nylon jacket, he walked into the lobby of a local business, and a loud explosive sound, like a large firecracker, erupted when he walked on the carpet. Burn marks began to appear on the carpet where his footsteps had singed it.

Firemen were called. They evacuated the building and, as a precaution, impounded Clewer's nylon jacket. Fire brigade official Henry Barton told Reuters news agency that Clewer's clothes carried an electrical charge of up to 30,000 volts, a level he called, only half in jest, quite shocking.

In an unrelated incident, a columnist for the *Sydney Morning Herald* newspaper reported in 1992 that he was literally thrown from his chair when he switched on his office computer. He had walked across synthetic carpet fibers while wearing synthetic clothing. The accumulated charge that had built up in his body and clothes got transferred into the electrical machinery, causing an explosive reaction and a painful zapping.

You probably have never generated explosive charges like these, but you may have experienced minor effects from electrostatic discharges. Naturally occurring static electricity builds up during the course of the day when wear synthetic fiber clothing, so when you touch a car door, a metal grocery cart, or even another person, you get a jolting electric shock. While these may seem like rare and relatively benign effects, a larger and more ominous health issue emerges from the scientific literature about electrostatic discharges caused by synthetic fiber clothing.

It's no secret that male fertility, as measured by sperm counts, has been in decline every decade since World War II, perhaps not coincidentally, since synthetic clothing has become a fixture in mainstream American wardrobes. Average sperm counts worldwide dropped 50 percent in the last half of the twentieth century, and according to the World Health Organization, up to 12 percent of all couples with women of childbearing age are now infertile. Environmental effects, such as endocrine disrupting synthetic chemicals, are certainly one cause of the infertility epidemic, but there is evidence that we also have synthetic clothing to blame.

It took putting polyester underpants on by a group of male dogs to establish the first scientific link between synthetic undergarments and infertility in human males. This 1993 study published in the medical journal *Urological Research* described how researchers put loose-fitting polyester underpants on twelve dogs over a period of twenty-four months, during which time their semen quality, testicular temperature, hormones, and testicular biopsies were examined. A second group of twelve dogs wore loose-fitting cotton underpants over the same period. Wearing polyester produced a degeneration of the testes and "significant decreases" in the sperm counts for all dogs in the first group. The dogs outfitted with cotton undergarments, by contrast, experienced no such reproductive side effects.

What could account for the effect of polyester undergarments and pants on fertility? The medical researchers in this study concluded: "It may be assumed that the electrostatic potentials generated by the polyester fabric play a role." In other words, polyester creates an electrostatic field around the crotch area of polyester wearers, and that can affect their sperm quality over time.

A year earlier another medical study, this one published in the journal *Archives of Andrology,* had tested the electrostatic potentials generated by various textile fabrics, including polyester. Twenty-one volunteers had been divided into three equal groups. The first group wore 100 percent polyester underpants, the second group wore a 50/50 polyester-cotton mix, and the third group wore 100 percent cotton. Over four days of wearing the various fabrics, an electrostatic kilovoltmeter measured each group's electrostatic field across the scrotal area. The cotton underpants created no electrostatic field but the polyester pants showed a high electrostatic charge, and the mixed polyester-cotton garments also generated a charge, but less so.

Four years later, in 1996, the same medical journal, *Archives of Andrology,* published a study that made the link between polyester and aberrations in male sexuality even more compelling. Fifty men were recruited and divided into four test groups to measure the effect of different types of textile underpants on sexual desire and the frequency of sexual activity. The underpants made of 100 percent polyester, a 50-50 polyester/cotton mix, 100 percent cotton, and 100 percent wool.

"Sexual behavior was assessed before and after six and twelve months of wearing the pants, and six months after their removal," wrote the study authors. "Behavioral response was rated as potent if the subject's penis became erect, entered the vagina, and ejaculated. The electrostatic potentials generated on the penis and scrotum were measured by an electrostatic kilovoltmeter."

At the end of the study period, it was found that the men who wore 100 percent polyester and the polyester-cotton mix underpants experienced "significantly reduced" sexual desire and sexual activity. Here is how the medical research team explained their findings: "The polyester-containing pants generated electrostatic potentials, which may induce electrostatic fields in the intrapenile structures and could explain the diminished sexual activity. The cotton and wool textiles did not generate electrostatic potentials. Thus, polyester underpants could have an injurious effect on human sexual activity."

There may be other factors at work as well. Natural cotton, even when tightly fitted, still enables the skin "to breathe," whereas synthetic clothing that fits tightly tends to trap body heat and encourages the skin to more readily absorb chemicals that are off gassed by the synthetic fibers.

A pioneering study of tight-fitting underwear and sperm quality in 1996, published in *The Lancet,* concluded that men who are trying to father a child shouldn't wear tight-fitting underwear of any sort because it can raise testes temperature to levels that interfere with sperm production.

Your common sense would be on target if it tells you that the genital area is the most sensitive part of the human body for chemical absorption. For men, the specific area of concern is the scrotum. Here's how a December 1989 article written by a New York University Medical School professor in *Cutis,* the dermatology medical journal, described the scrotal area's sensitivity: "The scrotum must be recognized as a skin area with remarkable permeability. It provides a unique percutaneous doorway for the entrance of drugs into the circulation and is thus uniquely susceptible to toxic and irritant agents."

Other medical authorities have estimated that the human scrotum may be twenty times more permeable than any other section of skin on the human body, yet little consideration seems to have been given by clothing manufacturers to this Achilles' heel for toxin absorption. Chemicals are routinely added to male infant and children's underpants, and to athletic supporters and tight-fitting synthetic underwear worn by boys and men. All of these garments rub against the scrotum. Add to that the presence of heat and the constrictive nature of these clothing items, and factors are in place to create a synergistic interaction that may further contribute to male infertility.

Stain-Resistant Clothing Can Disrupt Your Hormones

Clothes that are made to prevent stains by repelling grease and liquids carry an understandable appeal for many consumers. After all, you don't have to worry as much about being careful when you're a sloppy eater, and you don't have to worry about washing the clothes as often as normal. What you may need to worry about, however, is the toxicity of the perfluorooctanoic acid (PFOA) that helps clothing and other fabrics resist the stains of everyday living.

Thyroid disease was linked to PFOA exposure in a 2010 study published in the journal *Environmental Health Perspectives.* People with higher concentrations of PFOA in their blood were twice as likely to develop thyroid disease than people with lower concentrations. That finding was based on studying blood samples from 3,966 adults and comparing them to the incidence of thyroid disease.

This finding duplicated the results of previous animal studies that documented how the chemical compound can alter the mammalian thyroid hormone system. This system plays an essential role in maintaining your body's heart rate and regulating metabolism, body temperature, digestion, and other functions.

"There have long been suspicions that PFOA concentrations might be linked to changes in thyroid hormone levels," commented study author David Melzer, a professor of epidemiology and public health in Britain. "Our analysis shows that in the 'ordinary' adult population there is a solid statistical link between higher concentrations of PFOA in blood and thyroid disease."

Still another disturbing health study, this one published in a 2009 issue of *Human Reproduction* by a team of researchers from the UCLA School of Public Health, linked PFOA to infertility in women. By measuring PFOA levels in 1,240 women from the Danish National Birth Cohort at intervals between four and fourteen weeks of their pregnancies, the researchers discovered that the likelihood of infertility increased by 60 to 154 percent for women with the highest levels of PFOA in their blood, compared to women with the lowest levels. The menstrual cycles of the woman with the most PFOA also became irregular.

Higher PFOA levels also delay pregnancy, in those women who were eventually able to have a child.

An earlier human study had shown that PFOA may impair the growth of babies in the womb. Two epidemiological studies also uncovered evidence that PFOA can disrupt fetal growth. Researchers suspect that these stain-resistance chemicals can similarly affect men's sperm quality, which presents another layer of obstacles to highly industrialized nations that are trying to maintain their fertility and birth rates.

CHAPTER 4

We Are All Guinea Pigs

Men and women who join the ranks of our armed forces are aware that their lives might periodically be placed in jeopardy because they wear the uniform of their country. It's an occupational hazard. Wearing a uniform can turn them into a target. But what if the actual uniforms they wear each day as part of their military service hide potential threats to their long-term health? What if the safety of chemicals that are invisibly embedded in the uniform fabric is in doubt? Don't military men and women and those who care about them deserve to know the facts about any potential dangers?

Chemicals that wait silently to ambush human health can be just as elusive and deceptive as any foreign adversary. These chemicals were created to be protectors of our military personnel. They were incorporated into uniforms to make their lives easier and more comfortable. The problem is that these chemicals may inflict more damage than the military leadership that authorized them ever imagined possible. Their true nature and their actual effects on human health have never been fully investigated.

In a very real sense, our military personnel have been unknowing guinea pigs in tests that help to determine whether chemicals in clothing can have wider consumer applications for the civilian population. It's not a conspiracy. They're not being treated this way with malicious intent. It's simply a reflection of how institutions—be they government, military, or corporate business—make far-reaching assumptions about synthetic chemical safety, often based on shallow and incomplete research.

Beginning in 2010 the U.S. Department of Defense decreed that two types of chemicals—antifire and antiinsect—be added to military uniforms. Here is how the U.S. Army Center for Health Promotion and Preventive Medicine described the additives: "All deploying soldiers will be issued Flame-Resistant Army Combat Uniforms that have been factory treated with permethrin ... the factory treatment process uses special binders to ensure that enough permethrin is retained in (the uniforms) to protect against insect bites for the lifetime of the uniform."

Even after being laundered at least fifty times—the estimated combat life of a uniform—the fabric containing permethrin will retain its insect killing power. Even beyond the life of a uniform, permethrin will remain in the fabric because "only a very small amount of repellant will leave the uniform when laundered," according to the military health agency. As for disposal, the health agency informed military personnel that the uniforms treated with insecticide and flame retardants "can simply be deposited in the trash and require no special disposal process when the uniform is no longer serviceable." This advice was given without proper study and consideration of the impact of careless disposal on landfills, where the chemicals can seep into underlying groundwater resources.

Many disturbing questions are raised by these official instructions that were given to members of the armed forces and their families. Let's more closely examine the two types of chemicals—flame retardants and the insecticide permethrin—that have been added to clothing in a misguided though well-intentioned effort to keep our military personnel healthy and safe.

Let's begin with the flammability question and why the military started adding flame retardants to uniforms. That decision was partly in response to the fire dangers posed by most synthetic clothing sold in the civilian sector of the marketplace.

A "Burning Question" for the Troops

It took the burning disfigurement of numerous unfortunate U.S. Marines who were serving in Iraq to finally underscore just how dangerous the wearing of synthetic fabrics can be. Synthetic clothing made of polyester, acrylic, and nylon melts in the presence of high heat and fuses the materials to human skin. Here is how the Marine Corps publication, *Leatherneck,* described this horrible process in 2006: "Imagine a molten glob of melted plastic running down charred skin, oozing into your pores like a lava tattoo. That's your synthetic, designer T-shirt. Designed to keep people supercool in sweltering heat, man-made fabrics generally do just the opposite when the temperatures really soar. Expose them to fire and they often melt like birthday candles, seeping into the burnt flesh and making a bad injury even worse."

As an illustration of the dangers of synthetics, military medical officials pointed to a patient admitted to a medical facility at Camp Ramadi in Iraq. "We had a Marine with significant burn injuries covering around 70 percent of his body," reported Navy Commander Joseph Rappold, the chief medical officer. "His polyester shirt melted to his skin when the armored vehicle he was riding in struck an improvised explosive device. His injuries would not have been as severe had he not been wearing a polyester shirt."

In 2006, in response to the increasing number of severe burns associated with synthetic clothing, the commanding general of the Marines in Iraq ordered his troops to stop wearing synthetic fabrics any time they went off base. This ban extended to product lines made by Under Armour, Coolmax, and Nike, and included synthetic T-shirts, pants, boxer shorts, panties, and socks, which are all commonly sold in military clothing stores. A year earlier, a similar ban on synthetic clothing had gone into effect for military personnel working in aviation, fuel tank transport, and other hazardous duties that flash fires in which they would be vulnerable to that could melt chemical-laden fabrics.

To replace these "wicking fabrics," as synthetics came to be known in the military, officers recommended that 100 percent cotton clothing be worn when personnel were off base or on missions. But even Marines who never ventured off base were being warned by superiors that the use of synthetic clothing could be a dangerous risk to safety. Examples included incidents in which Marines had experienced electrical shocks while still on base. The shocks caused their synthetic clothing to begin smoking and discharging sparks.

A range of civilian professionals who commonly use synthetic clothing when in contact with high heat—from restaurant chefs to welders—need to be aware that they face many of the same dangers as military personnel. High flammability in synthetic clothing used by civilians may become an ever-greater health menace in the future as manufacturers compete to add more "functional" elements based on new chemical formulations.

Garment Flame Retardants Make Their Appearance

For decades firemen, race car drivers, astronauts, military pilots and others in hazardous professions have worn flame-retardant fibers with varying levels of thickness based on the risks they faced. Attempts to make clothing fire resistant began at least as far back as 1735, when a patent was filed in Britain for a chemical mixture of alum, ferrous sulfate, and borax that could be applied to fabrics. More chemical combinations were tried throughout the nineteenth century but failed to work properly because washing usually removed most or all of the fire-resistant chemicals. Not until 1912, when a chemist created a "non-flam" process with stannic oxide, did a practical application emerge that could withstand washing.

Additional research over subsequent decades, funded especially by the U.S. Army Quartermaster Corps, produced more durable and flame-resistant fabrics by chemically modifying cotton. For example, a chemical coating called Proban, which retains its effectiveness in fabric after up to thirty-five washings, was introduced by Westex, a U.S. firm.

Some of these blends were adopted by fire departments and by NASA for use in space suits during the early 1960s. By the early twenty-first century, with wars in Iraq and Afghanistan generating many burn injuries from improvised explosives, the U.S. military became the biggest buyer and user of flame-retardant fabrics.

Starting in 2007, flame-resistant uniforms became standard issue for U.S. troops in both Iraq and Afghanistan. The uniforms are made from a fabric called Nomex. This fiber product, first marketed by DuPont in 1967, resists high-temperature burning for about nine seconds, which was thought to be enough time for troops to either exit a burning vehicle or remove the fire-affected clothing. Military pilots had already been wearing flight suits composed of 92 percent Nomex blended with Kevlar threads as protection from cockpit fires.

With demand high for fire-retardant uniforms and civilian clothing, there was a virtual explosion of retardant clothing innovations, most of which used chemicals and chemical combinations that lacked any long-term safety testing. At least twenty-one different fire-retardant types of fabric are now being sold for use in both civilian and military clothing. To illustrate the attendant dangers of this trend, we describe an event that happened in Australia.

At the Ergon Energy plant in Queensland, Australia, the 3,400-strong workforce was outfitted with flame-retardant, Chinese-made uniforms during late August of 2008. Within a couple of weeks of wearing these new retardant uniforms, which cost $3.5 million, nearly two hundred employees began to suffer severe allergic reactions. Some workers were stricken with chronic vomiting, others broke out in blisters and complained of nausea, headaches, and other symptoms. When the uniforms were ironed, they released a yellow, bubbling substance that triggered other allergic reactions. Testing by chemists at an independent lab showed that the uniforms contained high levels of toxic chemicals, which was no big surprise given the severity of medical symptoms the workers had experienced.

Retardants Migrate to Affect Health

The effect of flame retardants on consumer health would disturb anyone who examines the evidence. When added to consumer products, such as sofa and chair fabric, retardant chemicals tend to migrate into the environment, especially into homes where the chemicals can easily be absorbed from dust by humans and animals and bioaccumulate in their body tissues and organs.

To measure the levels of brominated fire retardants accumulating in household dust, the Environmental Working Group (EWG) sampled dust in nine homes in eight states, from Florida to Oregon, in 2004. Here is how the EWG describes this category of retardants: "Like PCBs, their long-banned chemical relatives, the brominated fire retardants known as PBDEs (polybrominated diphenyl ethers) are persistent in the environment and bioaccumulate, building up in people's bodies over a lifetime. In minute doses they and other brominated fire retardants impair attention, learning, memory, and behavior in laboratory animals."

While two of three PBDE products, octa and penta, were removed from the market as health dangers in 2004, a third product called deca, which is used mostly in electronics, remained in use. The predominant type of retardant that EWG found in household dust was, in fact, deca, which over time breaks down into other toxic chemicals.

Previously, in 2003, EWG had measured the levels of retardants in the breast milk of U.S. mothers and found alarmingly high concentrations. Deca was detected in sixteen of twenty breast milk samples, which should be of concern to every parent since deca has proven to be toxic to lab animals that have been exposed to it during experiments.

We know next to nothing about the long-term health effects of newly created fire-retardant chemicals that are being added to clothing, which doesn't bode well for us since we are constantly finding out about new dangers associated with other consumer product retardants, many of which have been widely available in the marketplace for several decades.

A perceptive article in the *Globe and Mail* (Toronto) in August 2008, pointed out "no matter what flame retardant is used, it shows up in the environment." First up came the polychlorinated biphenyls, banned in the 1970s as a toxin to human and animal life, which were then replaced by PBDEs (polybrominated diphenyl ethers), which were even used in baby clothing. Those PBDEs also migrated and were bioaccumulating rapidly in distant wildlife such as whales living in the Arctic. (PBDEs attach to dust particles and blow in the wind for thousands of miles.)

Laboratory studies determined that PBDEs can cause a wide range of health problems—thyroid hormone disruption, brain damage, ADHD-like symptoms, and reproductive defects and other fertility problems. The forms of retardants that have been suspended from sale and distribution still show up in the environment and in human body tissues. They are quite resilient. A replacement for these suspended chemicals, called brominated phthalates, began appearing in household dust in 2009, demonstrating that each new generation of retardants migrates like the previous generations.

As the EWG noted in relation to retardants in consumer goods, a host of safety questions remain to be answered: Do some people absorb more retardants than others? Do they metabolize the chemicals differently once they are absorbed? Why do some people excrete the chemicals slowly, enabling the bioaccumulation to reach dangerous levels of toxicity? What happens when these chemicals synergize with other potentially toxic chemicals in the body? A lot of research on these cxhemicals remains to be done before we can even begin to pronounce them safe for human exposure.

Health Problems and Flame Retardants

- The category of retardants called PBDEs appears in the bodies of almost 100 percent of the U.S. population, based on findings from blood tests conducted by the U.S. Centers for Disease Control and Prevention *(Environmental Health Perspectives,* May 1, 2010).

• Two new chemical retardant replacements for toxic flame retardants in household products also leach into the environment, and have been detected in peregrine falcon eggs in California. This finding adds to mounting evidence that newly introduced retardants escape into the environment and persist there like all previous retardants have been seen to do (*Science News,* March 27, 2010).

• When breast milk samples were taken from more than three hundred North Carolina women, flame retardant contamination was found in three-quarters of them. The highest levels measured were in women twenty-five to twenty-nine years of age (*Environmental Health News,* Jan. 25, 2010).

• Retardants in household products contribute to fertility problems by lengthening the time it takes for women to get pregnant. Animal studies also show that PBDEs can influence ovulation and menstrual cycles (*Environmental Health News,* June 3, 2010).

• Children with higher concentrations of PBDEs in their umbilical cord blood at birth experience developmental effects, both physical and mental, within a few years. These include lower IQ scores (Columbia University study released via *EurekAlert,* Jan. 19, 2010).

Flame Resistant versus Flame Retardant

Though the terms are often used interchangeably by consumers, there is a slight difference between "flame resistant" and "flame retardant." Any fabric that resists being ignited, but tends to extinguish itself once on fire, qualifies as a flame-resistant garment. Wool is a good example.

By contrast, a flame retardant is any chemical substance applied to make a fabric resistant to fire and burning. Flame-retardant chemicals are either bonded into clothing fibers during the manufacturing process or applied as coatings to the finished fabrics.

The actual chemical composition for most of these fire retardants isn't known to the public because the chemical formulas are "proprietary" corporate trade secrets. This kind of secrecy is surprisingly common for chemical mixtures sold in the United States thanks to a legal loophole, as pointed out in a previous chapter. Under the 1976 Toxic Substances Control Act, chemical manufacturers are exempt from disclosing any product details that might harm their profits by giving competitors inside information.

As a result of this maddening secrecy, researchers who attempt to identify toxins that might be a threat to human health end up being thwarted in their disclosure efforts. A January 4, 2010, article in the *Washington Post,* revealed what happened to Duke University chemist Heather Stapleton, who had been trying for months to identify a mystery chemical that she had uncovered in household dust samples from Boston-area homes.

As the newspaper reported: "While attending a conference, she (Stapleton) happened to see the structure of a chemical she recognized as her mystery compound. The substance is a chemical in 'Firemaster 550,' a product made by Chemtura Corporation for use in furniture and other products as a substitute for a flame retardant the company quit making in 2004 because of health concerns. Stapleton found that Firemaster 550 contains an ingredient similar in structure to a chemical—di(2-ethylhexyl) phthalate, or DEHP—that Congress banned last year from children's products because it has been linked to reproductive problems and other health effects.

Chemtura keeps the ingredients of Firemaster 550 confidential, and contends that concerns about profits and competitiveness should outweigh concerns about safety and health. But as environmental scientist Susan Klosterhaus told the *Post:* "My concern is we're using chemicals and we have no idea what the long-term effects might be or whether or not they're harmful."

21 Fire-Retardant Materials Known to Be in Clothing

- Arselon (a Swedish company product)
- Carbon Foam
- Carbon X
- Dale Antiflame
- Indura (a Westex U.S. product)
- Kanox
- Kermel
- Kevlar
- Lenzing FR (a Rayon fire retardant)
- M5 fiber (a Magellan chemical company product)
- Mazic
- Modacrylic (a Solutia Inc. U.S. product and Kaneka Corp. Japan product)
- Nomex (a DuPont product)
- Nylon (coated)
- PBI
- Proban (a Westex U.S. product)
- Pyromex (a Toho Tenax Japanese product)
- Pyrovatex
- Technora (a Teijin company product of Japan)
- Teijinconex
- Twaron (a Dutch product)

A Killer Hides in Outdoor Clothing

What began in the 1980s as an attempt to protect military personnel from malaria and other insectborne diseases has created a widely pervasive problem in outdoor clothing. The practice of intentionally adding toxins to fabrics as an insect repellant is now commonplace throughout both the military and civilian clothing industries worldwide.

Permethrin became the insecticide of choice for use in clothing fabric to kill ticks, mosquitos, and black flies, and by all accounts, this carcinogen performs its killing duties with great efficiency and tenacity. Even after one hundred washings, according to clothing manufacturers, permethrin retains the ability to repel insects.

That might seem, at first, to be a wholly good thing. After all, any technique that effectively protects our soldiers from illness and disease would seem desirable. But what are the hidden costs to their health over time?

These questions are made all the more urgent by the increasing use of permethrin in outdoor clothing that is now being sold to people of all ages, the most vulnerable being children and pregnant women. Tommy Hilfiger markets a line of golf shorts and cotton polo shirts that are treated with permethrin, for example, while L.L. Bean sells shirts, hats, and hiking pants that are treated with it.

One of the first civilian clothing lines to feature permethrin was Buzz Off Insect Shield, which also introduced a line of kid's clothes that contains insecticide. As the National Coalition Against the Misuse of Pesticides in Washington, D.C., later reported, "The outdoor stores selling the clothing, including REI, EMS, and Hudson Trail Outfitters, appear to know very little about the pesticide contained in the clothing. Although permethrin is being described by Buzz Off's manufacturers as 'a man-made version of a repellant that occurs naturally in chrysanthemums,' in reality, permethrin is engineered to be much more toxic and persistent than natural pyrethrins."

"The new line of kid's clothing," continued an August 2, 2004, *Action Alert* from the pesticides watchdog group, "is particularly offensive as children are known to be more susceptible to the adverse effects of low-dose pesticide exposure. Animal studies have shown permethrin, in particular, to be more toxic to young children than adults and to potentially inhibit neonatal brain development."

Furthermore, Buzz Off's and similar insecticide-impregnated clothing was marketed without any warnings on the labels about the presence of a potentially toxic chemical. There was no indication of the effects on human health or the environment, and not even a caution that certain uses of the garments could result in greater health risks.

A portion of all permethrin on clothing comes off on the skin and is absorbed by the skin. If you sweat or swim while wearing the clothing, even more of the chemical will come off, and a portion will be absorbed. The longer you wear the clothing, the more insecticide you will absorb. But the labels issue no cautions or, indeed, any worthwhile information whatsoever about these conditions of use.

There is even the possibility that being exposed to sunlight while wearing permethrin clothing will corrupt the wearer's immune system, according to research by Virginia Tech Professor Steven D. Holladay and his toxicology co-researchers. "Nobody really knows at this point the risk that the clothes pose," Professor Holladay has been quoted as saying.

People of every age who have worn these garments are guinea pigs in a long-term, uncontrolled experiment. They never gave their consent to being guinea pigs, nor were they made aware of the risks they are subjecting themselves and their children to in the name of comfort.

Five Health Concerns About Outdoor Clothing

We have detected at least five potential problems with permethrin being attached to fibers in clothing, whether it's used in military uniforms or civilian outdoor wear:

1. No long-term safety testing has been done to determine the health effects of repeatedly wearing permethrin garments.
2. Skin absorption estimates for permethrin clothing made by manufacturers have probably been much too low.
3. Permethrin exposure from other common everyday sources hasn't been factored into the safety estimates for permethrin clothing.
4. The additive or synergistic effects of permethrin mixing with flame retardants in the fabric or on the skin, or mixing with other chemicals associated with clothing manufacturing, are potential hazards in need of further study.
5. The impact on ecosystems from the disposal of used permethrin clothing hasn't been properly evaluated.

Let's examine each of these concerns, one by one, in more detail.

Concerns 1 and 2: Long-term safety and skin absorption.

To illustrate how little, if any, long-term safety testing or continual monitoring has been done on permethrin garments to assess potential threats to health, we describe the skin absorption study estimates that have been made over the years. Manufacturers and military health officials have always contended that the levels of permethrin that are absorbed from clothing through the skin are so low (or nonexistent) as to render any health considerations moot. Let's look at their claim that permethrin isn't easily absorbed by human skin.

Using low absorption level estimates as a baseline, a panel of toxicologists, called the Subcommittee to Review Permethrin Toxicity from Military Uniforms, concluded in 2003 that "exposure to permethrin from wearing treated uniforms is unlikely to cause harmful effects to fetuses or newborns." The U.S. Environmental Protection Agency adopted these findings as a rationale for approving the commercial sale of permethrin-treated outdoor clothing for use by children and pregnant women.

Should we now feel safer about insecticide in our clothing because of these determinations? A study from Germany, done in 2010, provides us with part of the answer. A team of toxicology researchers from the University Medical Center of the Johannes Gutenberg University decided to examine the exposure and health risks that can arise from wearing permethrin-impregnated clothing, since the German military was also equipping its personnel with permethrin-impregnated battle dress uniforms (Rossbach 2010).

A controlled trial was conducted with a study group of 187 volunteers, of which a subgroup of eighty-six people wore the permethrin uniforms for twenty-eight days. The other people in the control group wore untreated clothing. Internal exposure to permethrin was assessed by measuring all of the subject's urinary permethrin metabolites on days 0, 14, and 28, and after the termination of the study.

As expected, those who wore the untreated clothing showed permethrin exposure levels similar to that of the general German population. However, in the participants who wore the permethrin-treated-uniforms, the study authors measured "considerably higher metabolite concentrations ... due to these results, a substantial uptake of permethrin from impregnated battle dress uniforms has to be assumed." In other words, not only was permethrin readily absorbed by the skin, the levels of permethrin being absorbed from fabric exposure were much higher than anyone ever suspected.

Even in the face of this finding, the study authors didn't believe health impairments were likely because the levels failed to exceed a maximum permethrin daily uptake standard that had been established by other toxicologists. Assuming this daily exposure level of safety is accurate, this and other studies ignore the *long-term* impact of absorbing permethrin every day for months and even years on end. This German study only lasted one month. How much permethrin builds up in fat tissue and body organs over longer periods of time? Mainstream toxicologists don't seem to know.

Duke University toxicology researchers have published a series of studies over the past decade that examine permethrin and its additive or synergistic effects when it is used in combination with other chemicals. Study team leader Dr. Mohammed Abou-Donia has identified three big health problems with wearing permethrin-impregnated clothing: (1) prolonged exposure risks from wearing such clothing; (2) the combined exposure risks when permethrin is used with DEET and other chemical agents; (3) certain segments of the population, such as pregnant women, young children, and the elderly, have increased sensitivity to permethrin, which makes them more at risk for health impairments.

"There is an urgent need for studies to document the safety of (permethrin) and related chemicals," Dr. Abou-Donia was quoted as saying after publication of his team's studies. "Right now we just don't have enough."

Concern 3: Permethrin exposure from other everyday sources hasn't been factored into the safety estimates for permethrin clothing.

Permethrin-soaked clothes are not the only source of large exposures to the insecticide. The chemical is found in many personal-size mosquito sprays and commonly shows up in residential bug sprays that are used by exterminators. It appears in lice shampoos for pets and people, along with flea dips and household foggers. It kills insects by disrupting their nervous systems.

The daily maximum exposure level for safety with permethrin can be exceeded from the combined effects of absorbing it from clothing and a person's proximity to mosquito repellants being used, especially if the repellants are released within confined spaces, as would be the case with the lice and flea products.

For persons whose jobs involve handling permethrin, there is already a well-documented three-fold increase in the risk for developing Parkinson's disease. A September 2009 study published in the *Archives of Neurology* compared 519 people with Parkinson's to 511 people without, and determined that those whose jobs involved exposure to the insecticide tripled their risk for developing the disease compared to those reporting no exposure to the chemical agent.

Other studies have linked permethrin exposure to cancer, endocrine system disruption, kidney and liver damage, and a range of developmental and reproductive disorders. The EPA identifies it as moderately toxic and labels it a restricted use category of pesticide.

Concern 4: The additive and synergistic effects of permethrin that

is combined with other chemicals are a potential health hazard.

In daily life we absorb minute quantities of dozens—perhaps hundreds—of chemicals that leach from our clothes, personal care products, foods, and the surrounding environment. When people wear permethrin-coated clothing, for instance, they often seek additional protection from irritating insects by applying other bug killers to their skin and clothes.

No long-term studies have been done to test what happens when permethrin and flame retardants from fabric mix on skin, so we don't know yet whether the resulting synergistic effects will produce serious health problems. But studies on the additive and synergistic effects of permethrin have been conducted with other pesticides, such as DEET, and the results should be a bright red warning flag for manufacturers, government regulators, and all consumers.

Beginning in 2001, a series of experiments performed by a Duke University team of pharmacology researchers uncovered evidence that permethrin interacts with DEET and other chemical agents to produce severe health problems in lab animals. There was even evidence that linked DEET and permethrin to the range of health symptoms known as Gulf War Syndrome. Chronic headaches, memory loss, fatigue, and joint pain were experienced by thousands of veterans from the first Persian Gulf War. This happened to be the first conflict in which military personnel used permethrin and DEET on their clothing and skin in combination—based on military health service advice—to ward off sand flies and other desert pests.

Using the same doses of permethrin and DEET used by military personnel and the same routes of body exposure, Dr. Mohammed Abou-Donia and his Duke University research team documented neurological damage in their lab animals that produced learning and memory dysfunction and a host of motor disorders. The researchers noted that when DEET is applied to skin that is already exposed to permethrin-clothing, absorption of permethrin into the bloodstream is accelerated. This is a phenomenon that the EPA apparently never took into consideration in approving its use, nor had the agency considered the synergistic effects of these and other chemicals acting together when approval was made.

These considerations gain ever-greater importance when we consider how often the permethrin in outdoor clothing comes into contact with DEET and other bug sprays and ointments. Clothing labels for some of the insecticide clothing brands even specifically advise wearers to use the clothes "in conjunction with an insect repellent registered for direct application to skin." The idea seems to be that slathering on more insecticide is always better than not using enough.

"Children in particular are at risk," cautions Professor Abou-Dania. "Their skin more readily absorbs it, and it more potently affects their developing nervous systems." At first, the symptoms of exposure might be subtle—slight muscle weakness, attention disruption, fatigue—but over time full-blown health problems could develop.

To provide a glimpse at the potential dangers of using permethrin by itself, or mixing it with other substances on your skin, we summarize findings from just a few alarming studies:

- Permethrin in combination with one or more other pesticides "significantly decreased" sperm quality, affecting reproduction in lab animals that were exposed to their additive effects (Perobelli 2010).
- Longer-term effects of permethrin on lab animal health was tested over sixty days. Daily treatment on the skin for that period resulted in hormone disruption, reproductive abnormalities, and other problems (Issam 2010).
- When permethrin was applied to the skin of lab rats, both by itself and combined with DEET or another pesticide, malathion, "all behavioral measures were impaired" and exposure induced "neuronal degeneration in the brain" (Abdel-Rahman 2004).
- To assess permethrin and other insecticide exposure levels, 5,046 urine samples were taken from U.S. residents. Permethrin showed up in more than 70 percent of the samples, with children having higher levels of absorption than adults, prompting the nine study authors from the U.S.

Centers for Disease Control and Prevention to warn that permethrin is "an acute neurotoxicant" (Barr 2010).

Concern 5: The impact of permethrin on ecosystems.

Many studies have documented that permethrin is toxic to fish and other aquatic life. This occurs even at low exposure levels.

A June 2006 advisory posted by the EPA states: "Permethrin is highly toxic to both freshwater and estuarine aquatic organisms," and "poses chronic risks." Also, "Toxicity data show that the compound is highly toxic to honeybees, as well as other beneficial insects."

Once released, the insecticide also persists in the environment, building up in creek and river sediments and bioaccumulating in bottom-dwelling fish and shellfish, some of which pass their toxic burden on to the humans who catch and then consume them.

When people swim in or wash permethrin-treated clothing, they release the chemical into the waterways. When municipal water treatment plants recycle the same water, the permethrin and many other chemicals cannot all be removed—the treatment plants aren't technologically advanced enough—so consumers end up drinking, bathing in, and cooking with this tainted water. As that old saying informs us, "What goes around comes around."

In a May 2009 website posting, the U.S. Army Center for Health Promotion and Preventive Medicine advises all members of the armed forces that "permethrin factory-treated flame-retardant clothing can simply be deposited in the trash and requires no special disposal process when the uniform is no longer serviceable." Clearly, the military is acting with reckless disregard for the health and environmental consequences of permethrin use.

CHAPTER 5

Fabric Care That Creates Toxins

Which Toxins Are You Washing Your Clothes In?

Most people never seem to give a passing thought to how their clothes are maintained, nor do they question whether the products they use each week create problems for their own health, much less for planetary health. How we choose to care for our clothes mirrors the broader issues of how we care our bodies and for the environment.

How often do you reflexively pick up a box or bottle of laundry detergent and make your buying decision based solely on its price, its reputation for effectiveness, or your own shopping habits? Most people never stop to consider that the seemingly simple choice about which detergent to buy can have broader implications. Since the average American family launders about three hundred loads of clothes each year, according to surveys done by Procter & Gamble, the laundry products we choose have a huge potential impact on our personal and collective well-being.

Finding out what chemicals are really in your laundry detergent and what effect they may be having requires some detective work. Detergent manufacturers aren't mandated by law to list ingredients on labels, which is an exemption granted to them under trade secrecy laws to protect their formulations from competitors. The information you will find on product labels is put there to give consumers a false sense of security about safety and commonly uses generic language such as "Ingredients include surfactants." "Surfactant" is just another term for detergent, and there are a wide variety of these cleansers in use.

Most major manufacturers of detergents have phased out phosphates, which remove hard water minerals to increase product effectiveness and prevent dirt from settling back onto clothes during the washing cycle. This action by manufacturers came in response to phosphate bans that were enacted by some state governments. The bans came about because the phosphates, once released back into the environment, stimulated explosive growth of undesirable plants that endanger sensitive ecosystems.

As an alternative to phosphates, detergent companies created numerous synthetic compounds that may exact an even greater toll. Research conducted by various environmental groups and by Dr. Samuel Epstein, an eminent toxicologist and founder of the Cancer Prevention Coalition, identified some of the new surfactants in laundry soap and uncovered the health consequences of exposure to these chemicals:

- Diethanolamine and triethanolamine are synthetic surfactants that were designed to neutralize acids, but they are carcinogens or can react with other chemicals to form nitrosamines, a family of carcinogens. They are slow to biodegrade and thus persist in the environment. They can also be found in many shampoos and conditioners.
- EDTA (ethylenediaminetraacetic acid) is used to reduce water hardness, and this compound can disrupt the hormones of humans and wildlife. Once released into the environment, it doesn't biodegrade easily and can dissolve toxic heavy metals that are trapped in underwater sediments so these toxins can re-enter the food chain. EDTA also appears in shampoos and other products as a "penetration enhancer" that is designed to allow others chemicals to penetrate more deeply.
- PEG (polyethylene glycol) is made from ethylene oxide, a potent carcinogen. Once in the environment, PEG is slow to biodegrade and has unknown consequences for wildlife. PEG is also commonly found in shampoos and conditioners.
- Quaternium-15 is a surfactant and disinfectant that releases formaldehyde, a potent carcinogen, and it's also an allergen that is often contaminated with DEA, still another carcinogen. This compound can also be found as a preservative in skin lotions, shampoos, and other products.

As if this wasn't enough to be concerned about, conventional detergents increasingly contain chemicals known as "optical brighteners." These are designed to make laundered clothes appear brighter and whiter, but they can cause allergic reactions in humans and can be toxic to fish once they are released into the environment with laundry wastewater. You probably won't find these chemicals identified on any product labels, though you should be alerted to their presence when you see a product claiming to "brighten" your clothing.

An analysis of laundry wastewater, both the industrial variety and that from public laundromats, was performed a few years ago by the Environmental Working Group (EWG). They detected that a range of hormone-disrupting contaminants was being released. Phthalates, used to stabilize fragrances, are human hormone disruptive chemicals that are commonly added to detergents and other cleaning products. Phthalates were detected in wastewater from four of the four laundries tested. This family of chemicals accumulates swiftly in the body tissues and blood of human beings, a finding that so alarmed the European Union that in 2005 it banned the use of most phthalates in products sold throughout Europe.

Another chemical found in the laundry wastewater by the EWG was triclosan, which is added as an antibacterial agent in detergents and is a chemical known to be toxic to liver functioning. Triclosan persists in both human bodies and the environment, bioaccumulating up the food chain. It has also been documented to play a role in reducing human resistance to antibiotics, which has helped stimulate the development of "superbug" bacteria.

Scented Laundry Products Release Toxins

Six top-selling laundry products were tested by University of Washington researchers, and each one was found to release "at least one chemical regulated as toxic or hazardous under federal laws, but none of those chemicals were listed on the product labels," reported *Science Daily* in a July 24, 2008, issue.

After hearing people complain that the scent from laundry products made them feel sick, Professor of Environmental Engineering Anne Steinemann decided to analyze the products to determine which chemicals were causing the health effects. "I was surprised by both the number and the potential toxicity of the chemicals that were found," Steinemann admitted to the magazine. Among the noxious chemicals she found were acetone, limonene, acetaldehyde, chloromethane, and 1,4-dioxane.

"Nearly one hundred volatile organic compounds were emitted from these six products, and none were listed on any product label. Plus, five of the six products emitted one or more carcinogenic 'hazardous air pollutants,' which are considered by the Environmental Protection Agency to have no safe exposure level," Steinemann revealed.

The products she analyzed included a dryer sheet, a fabric softener, and a detergent. "Be careful if you buy products with fragrance, because you really don't know what's in them," she warned. She urged consumers to buy only fragrance-free versions of laundry products. Her study, which was published in the journal *Environmental Impact Assessment Review,* didn't reveal the brand-names of the six products that her lab tested.

Previous to these study results, the European Union had enacted legislation requiring products to list the presence of twenty-six fragrance chemicals when they exceed designated levels in cosmetic products and detergents. No similar regulations exist in the United States and many other countries.

Beware of Chemical Fabric Softeners

Softeners may seem like a miracle product for keeping clothing comfortable for daily wear, but the downside of using these products is that you're allowing your skin and lungs to come into contact with some nasty toxins that "just keep on giving."

Still another survey of U.S. households done by Procter & Gamble in 2006 (whose results were shared with the U.S. Consumer Product Safety Commission) found that 71 percent of those surveyed use some form of fabric softener, with the most common forms for home laundering being liquid softeners (purchased by 42 percent of U.S. households) and dryer sheet softeners (used by 49 percent of households.) As you probably know, dryer sheet softeners have antistatic properties. Many households were found to be using both forms of softeners, with a rinse cycle softener followed by a dryer sheet for the same laundry load. This means that most Americans come into weekly contact with the chemicals that make up softener ingredients.

These chemicals include toxins like chloroform, benzyl acetate, pentane, and compounds that release formaldehyde. Whether used in liquid form or dryer sheets, the softeners leave chemical residues in your clothing by design, so they continually give off molecules. You breathe in the chemical fumes, especially after the treated clothes are heated in the dryer, and you absorb some of the residue through your skin when wearing the treated clothes.

Alison Petten, a Canadian registered nurse who works with the Environmental Health Association of Nova Scotia, has studied the health impacts of fabric softeners and their ingredients. She said "The ingredients in fabric softeners can irritate skin and cause asthma-like symptoms. I have seen marked improvements in clients with psoriasis, eczema, asthma, and migraines when they stopped using chemical fabric softeners. Others have told me that their irritable bowel syndrome and arthritis improved when they cut chemical fabric softeners out of their laundry routine. A lot of people don't make the connection that the chemicals that we breathe, and those we absorb through the skin, get into the bloodstream and can affect every organ and system in the body."

The role of chemical synergies in triggering health problems isn't understood by most ordinary consumers, or by many toxicologists and physicians, for that matter. As we indicated earlier, when two or more chemicals are combined in a product, or in the human body, they can sometimes produce toxic effects that are much more powerful than any one chemical can generate on its own.

24 Fragrance Allergens in Detergents to Avoid

Product ingredient labels usually don't identify the fragrance chemicals used to scent detergents (and through washing, your clothes) because no law in the United States requires them to be revealed. Fragrances in mainstream conventional detergents are made from petroleum, which means they don't biodegrade easily in the environment, can be toxic to fish and mammals, and can cause allergies and irritation in humans. Toluene, a common chemical in fragrances, is known to cause reproductive abnormalities and cancer in lab animals.

European Union standards for fragrance allergens in detergents and other products require clear product labeling so that fragrance-sensitive consumers can make informed choices about the products they purchase. No such labeling requirements exist in the United States Here are twenty-four common fragrances that are added to detergents, based on a list published in a July 2006 article in the journal *Contact Dermatitis.* (Conservative estimates are that 10 percent of the fragrance allergen on washed fabrics will be transferred to human skin when the fabrics are worn.)

- Amyl cinnamic aldehyde
- Cinnamic alcohol
- Cinnamic aldehyde (also commonly appears as an allergen in perfumes)
- Eugenol (also commonly appears as an allergen in perfumes)
- Geraniol (also commonly appears as an allergen in perfumes)
- Hydroxycitronella
- Isoeugenol (also commonly appears as an allergen in perfumes)
- Amyl cinnamic alcohol
- Anisyl alcohol
- Benzyl alcohol (also appears as an allergen in cosmetics)
- Benzyl benzoate (also commonly appears as an allergen in perfumes)
- Benzyl cinnamate (also commonly appears as an allergen in perfumes)

- Benzyl salicylate (also commonly appears as an allergen in perfumes)
- Citral (also commonly appears as an allergen in perfumes)
- Citronellol (also commonly appears as an allergen in perfumes)
- Coumarin (also commonly appears as an allergen in perfumes)
- Farnesol (also commonly appears as an allergen in perfumes)
- Gamma methyl ionone
- Hexyl cinnamic aldehyde
- Lilial
- d-Limonene (also listed as a carcinogen by the National Toxicology Program)
- Linalool (also commonly appears as an allergen in perfumes)
- Lyral (HMPCC)
- Methyl heptine carbonate

A pioneering study done in 1998, which examined the synergies produced by fragrance chemicals that are allergens, illustrates the dimensions of the synergy problem facing chemical manufacturers, the health-care industry, and all consumers who buy and use synthetics. Authored by five researchers and published in the *British Journal of Dermatology,* this University of Copenhagen (Denmark) study tested two groups of eczema patients. One group of eighteen patients had a contact allergy to two fragrance substances, the other control group was allergic to only one of the fragrances. Three separate allergy tests were conducted on both groups.

The researchers reported these results: "It was found that the combination of two allergens in individuals allergic to both substances had a synergistic effect ... the two allergens elicited responses as if the doses were three to four times higher than those actually used ... the synergistic effect demonstrated is likely to apply to other contact allergens as well..."

That study and its conclusions support a key theme in this book, *Killer Clothes.* It's not just the single doses of chemicals we absorb from synthetic clothing and clothing care products that should concern us—it's the cumulative doses that are interacting with each other and additional chemicals that are absorbed from cosmetics and personal care products that, taken together, might trigger synergies that produce serious health consequences. This means your body burden of synthetic chemicals, which is stored in your body fat and organs, needs to be reduced whenever possible, or at least not added to. Therefore, you must pay close attention to the total volume of chemicals you place into contact with your skin.

The Dry Cleaning Chemical That's a Killer

If you've ever taken clothes home from a dry cleaner and immediately tore open the plastic bags to extract the garments, you know how the clothes emit a chemical odor that you can't help but inhale. That's the residue of perchloroethylene, or Perc for short, the chemical solvent used by three-fourths of dry cleaning businesses in the United States.

While Perc is considered to be an efficient cleaning agent for clothing, it's also highly toxic and responsible for a wide range of well-documented harmful effects on human health. The International Association for Research on Cancer calls Perc a probable carcinogen based on animal testing and research studies going back three decades in *Environmental Health Perspectives* and other medical science journals. The studies have outlined Perc's many negative effects on health. These occur when it is inhaled or comes into contact with skin.

Environmental Health Professor Helen Suh MacIntosh of Harvard University has described how studies have found that Perc exposure increases a person's risk of bladder, esophageal, and cervical cancer; eye, nose, throat, and skin irritations; and even reduced fertility. She writes, "Low levels of perchloroethylene can be present in your indoor air, as any perchloroethylene that was not removed in the dry cleaning process will be on your clothes that you bring home. Once at home, the perchloroethylene will leave your clothes and go into the air."

Chemical manufacturers and the dry cleaning industry claim that the tiny amounts of Perc you may absorb through your lungs or skin from contact with dry cleaned clothes represent a negligible threat to human health and little danger to the environment. These claims weren't reassuring to regulators and health authorities in California, where the use of Perc was banned in 3,400 dry cleaning businesses by the end of 2010. The ban occurred after investigators found that the solvent had contaminated at least one in every ten of the state's water wells.

This finding about Perc contamination of water wells serves to underscore an uncomfortable fact about Perc—once released from clothing or from dry cleaning machinery, it persists in ecosystems, and once absorbed by the human body, it persists in body fat and organs. Perc has been tightly regulated in European countries, where policing of toxic chemicals that pose a threat to human health has been much more rigorous than in the United States.

Choose Nontoxic Cleaning Methods

Detergents were designed to lower the surface tension of water to make it interact with dirt and stains on clothing, separating the grime from the fabric. Petrochemical detergents do this effectively, but as we've pointed out, their use results in a range of unintended consequences.

You have a variety of alternatives to choose from when you decide to break free from dependence on toxic cleaning agents. You can purchase nontoxic laundry detergents created by green technology, or you can make your own safe cleaning mixtures.

Soap nuts are a type of dried berry that, like regular detergents, interact with water to produce cleansing actions on fabric. Sold at health food stores, these dried fruits come from a tree native to Asia. The website buysoapnuts.com also sells this easy-to-use product at affordable prices. The nuts can be used two or three times each and are 100 percent biodegradable.

Another natural cleaning agent can be found online at www.lifenatural.com. These special magnets go into the washing machine along with your load of laundry and help to remove grime from garments again and again, since the magnets never need to be replaced.

Finally, you can create your own laundry detergent at home with a few simple and inexpensive ingredients. Take two cups of grated gentle soap, such as Dr. Bronner's, and mix it well with one cup of washing soda and one cup of borax. Add one-fourth cup of this mixture to each load of laundry. Splash in a cup of white vinegar during the rinse cycle to brighten the appearance of the clothes.

CHAPTER 6

Dressing Yourself and Others Safely

Why Natural Fibers Are Safer

We need to take responsibility for our personal health and safety, as well as for the health of the people in our lives that depend on us for guidance and the exercise of good judgment. In the following chapter you will find positive advice about how to make buying decisions that will empower you personally, even as you help to protect the natural environment from the residue of our potentially toxic actions. The first priority is choosing natural fibers.

Your Most Common Natural Fiber Options:

Cotton. Of the thirty-nine species that grow worldwide, only four have been domesticated, the most common today being *G. hirsutum,* which was first grown in Central America by tribal societies. Cotton fragments from 5000BC have turned up in archaeological digs in Pakistan and Mexico. Today, cotton remains the "king" of textiles. Over the past decade the popularity of organic cotton (grown without pesticides) has increased, but still accounts for less than one percent of worldwide cotton production.

Flax. This fiber plant grows to a height of four feet and is considered one of nature's strongest fibers. Archaeologists have found evidence of its use in clothing going back to prehistoric times in the Near East. Later cultivation occurred in ancient Egypt, classical Greece, and imperial Rome. The plant is best known as the source of linen, which was used in its finest form to wrap the mummies of Egyptian pharaohs.

Hemp. Processed like flax, the hemp plant is versatile and hardy. It grows without any need for fungicides, herbicides, or pesticides because it's naturally insect resistant. Hemp was the original fabric for Levi's jeans before the company made a switch to cotton. Hemp cloth has made a comeback in T-shirts and other apparel over the past decade, especially among young people in the United States. Half of the world's hemp supply is grown in China. Its fibers are said to be four times stronger than cotton. In contrast to another variety of hemp known as marijuana, this species of hemp has no psychoactive properties.

Silk. Known as the "queen of fabrics," silk was first developed in ancient China, where for generations only royalty was allowed to wear it. It's produced by the larvae of a moth species that feeds on the leaves of the white mulberry tree. For about two thousand years the Chinese kept the methods used in collecting and weaving silk a closely guarded secret, until two priests smuggled some silkworm eggs to Constantinople in about 555 AD. Today's common silkworm doesn't exist in the wild and is bred only in domesticated silk farms. Nearly a dozen types of silk fabrics have emerged over the centuries, including brocade, chiffon, damask, and velvet. The use of synthetic dyes should be a concern for those who wear silk clothing.

Wool. Sheep's wool has provided humans with warm clothing for thousands of years, dating back to the first domestication of animals. Today, most commercially grown wool is contaminated with chemicals, such as pesticides used to kill parasites on the sheep. Organic wool is becoming more common, with New Mexico providing about 80 percent of U.S.-certified organic wool.

Less Common Natural Fiber Options

Alpaca. Found mainly in the Andes mountains of South America, this member of the camelid family has two distinct types of hair. Huacayo alpacas produce short, dense, soft fibers; Suri alpacas produce straight, silklike hairs. Both fibers are used to make luxury fabrics.

Angora. China produces most of the world's angora rabbit wool, followed by Argentina and Chile. Angora is a soft and fine fiber that is removed from the rabbit by shearing or combing every three months. It is used in high-quality knit wear.

Camel. Mongolia produces the highest-quality camel hair fibers. There are two types: a coarse outer hair and a fine inner down. White fleece is rare, the most common color is reddish brown. Camels's wool is used in sportswear, overcoats, and topcoats.

Cashmere. China is the world's largest producer of raw cashmere, which is shorn from the Kashmir goat. The hair fibers have strong insulation qualities but are soft to the touch. Most cashmere garments are sold in Europe, the United States, and Japan.

Mohair. The Angora goat is indigenous to Turkey, and its white, fine, and silky fiber is known for providing warmth in the winter. Yet it is so versatile that it's cool enough for the humidity of summer. The fiber is found in knitting yarn and is often combined with wool.

Ramie. This flowering plant is native to East Asia and is considered one of the strongest natural fibers. Its bark has been used for thousands of years in thread and twine and is spun into a grass cloth that is sometimes called "chinese linen." It's often blended with wool or cotton.

Saluyot. This is a relatively new entrant on the world's natural textile stage. Saluyot and water hyacinth plants grow everywhere in the Philippines, where their fibers are made into yarn for apparel. Saluyot is valued for the fineness of its fibers and its tensile strength. The Philippines grow about thirty useful natural fiber crops, including abaca, ramie, coconut coir, banana, and other leaf and plant fibers.

What Makes Organic Cotton Superior

Until the twentieth century the world's cotton production was entirely natural and organic, but by the end of that century, as synthetic chemicals came to dominate the marketplace, cotton crops accounted for about 10 percent of all the planet's pesticide usage and around 25 percent of all insecticides used. To put that toxic burden into human terms, the Organic Trade Association estimates that a single nonorganic cotton T-shirt is the product of one-third pound of pesticides and chemical fertilizers.

Over the past decade organic cotton made a comeback among producers and consumers owing to widening concerns about the impact of pesticides and insecticides on human health and the environment. You can now readily find organic cotton in all types of clothing, from casual to high fashion; in absorbent diapers, towels, bedding, and cushions; and even in personal care products, such as cotton swabs and tampons.

Patagonia is a California-based maker of casual and outdoor clothing that began using 100 percent organic fibers in all of its products in 1996. Larger manufacturers slowly followed suit. Nike added a blend of organic cotton to twenty million of its T-shirts, and Levi's purchased 330,000 pounds of organic cotton for making its 501 jeans. Most of these companies made business decisions that factored in the environmental costs of using toxic chemicals. "We are trying to use our company to bring environmental responsibility to the business dialogue," a spokeswoman for Patagonia, Lu Setnicka, told the Knight Ridder newspaper chain. "We know that other companies and farmers are listening."

6 Good Reasons to Choose Organic Natural Fibers

1. Eco-friendly and health-friendly organic fibers are grown and organic clothing is produced without the use of pesticides, herbicides, fungicides, genetic modifications, or other substances and processes that pose a danger to human health or the environment.
2. Nonorganic and synthetic fibers, by contrast, release chemicals and dyes during production and manufacturing that damage fragile ecosystems and harm wildlife.
3. Organic natural fibers are recyclable and biodegradable, whereas nonorganics and synthetics don't easily biodegrade and tend to accumulate in landfills, which poses a disposal problem for future generations.
4. Because organic fibers aren't degraded by chemicals during growing and processing, clothing made from these fibers is stronger than nonorganics and has a longer lifespan.

5. Natural organic fabrics are more absorbable and breathable for your skin than nonorganic and synthetic clothing. See for yourself by comparing how organic cotton feels against your skin on a hot and humid day as opposed to polyester or other synthetic blends.

6. Natural organic fibers don't release toxic fumes from chemicals when you wear them, whereas nonorganic synthetics off gas minute amounts of chemicals, which you then absorb through your skin and lungs.

One of the more established organic cotton farms is owned by Claude and Linda Sheppard of Chowchilla, California. They switched from chemical farming to organic farming in 1992, when Linda became pregnant and expressed concerns about her exposure to pesticides. They discovered that the organic cotton yields at harvest time on their 550 acres were the same as in the previous year, when they had used chemicals. "We were really amazed at how well it worked," Claude Sheppard told a *Fresno Bee* newspaper reporter. "After that, we stopped using all commercial fertilizers and herbicides. We ended up going completely organic."

When you purchase and wear organic cotton clothing, you not only benefit directly from its superior comfort and durability, you also help to minimize the harm to your health and the planet's ecosystems.

From seed preparation to weed control and harvesting, organic growing methods have proven to be safer because they don't rely on toxic chemicals. Following are some key differences between organic and conventional growing methods:

Seed preparation. Organic cotton farmers use seeds that are untreated by fungicides and insecticides and never use genetically modified seeds; none of this is true with conventional cotton farming.

Soil and water impacts. Organic cotton relies on crop rotation and water retention in the soil by adding organic matter; conventional cotton farming requires intensive irrigation to go with the application of synthetic fertilizers to the soil.

Weed control. Cultivation and hand-removal techniques control weeds in organic farming; conventional growers apply herbicides to thwart weed germination, and more herbicides are applied to kill weeds that survive.

Pest control. Beneficial insects and natural biological practices are used in organic farming to control pests; nonorganic cotton producers commonly use insecticides and pesticides, often by aerial spraying. Five of the more common pesticides are known carcinogens.

Harvesting. The site aboutorganiccotton.org points out that organic cotton harvests rely on seasonal freezes or water management for defoliation; nonorganic farming practices use toxic chemicals to defoliate cotton plants.

Hemp Makes Another Comeback

Even a casual review of the history of hemp fabric reveals it to be one of the most versatile and persistent fiber crops. Hemp was banned in the United States during the twentieth century because of an unfair association with its psychoactive cousin. However, it has made a comeback in the marketplace thanks to the agricultural policies of more enlightened countries.

Hemp fabrics have been in use among diverse cultures throughout the world for thousands of years. It is one of the few plants whose roots, stalks, leaf, flower, and seeds can all be used. Products such as food, medicine, writing paper, and lamp oil are made of hemp, which has hundreds of uses. For at least two thousand years most of the sailcloth and rigging lines used by seagoing vessels came from hemp.

One of the first large-scale uses of hemp for clothing in the United States came during the Revolutionary War of 1776, when General George Washington's army wore uniforms made from the plant, which happened to be a crop that Washington grew on his plantation, as did Thomas Jefferson. The first official flag of the thirteen states that flew over the U.S. Capitol was made of hemp fabric, as was the paper on which Jefferson and others wrote the first and second drafts of the Declaration of Independence.

Though the hemp that is used to make fabric contains little or no THC (the psychoactive ingredient in its cousin, marijuana), the plant still got caught up in the prohibition fever that gripped the United States during the 1930s. Growing hemp or even importing hemp products became a federal crime. The hemp industry believed the real motive behind prohibition was that hemp had become a competitive threat to the emerging synthetic fibers industry and the already established wood products industry. The ban on hemp cultivation was lifted briefly during World War II. While growing hemp crops remains strictly regulated in the United States, some relaxation on the importation of hemp products has occurred.

Beginning in the late 1980s, hemp garments began to be imported into the United States from China and other countries that had continued growing hemp and creating new products from it. Canada and China have since become two of the biggest suppliers to the U.S. market. Now hemp can be purchased in a wide variety of apparel options, including shoes, diapers, pants, shirts, and every other kind of garment.

What makes this plant so useful and valuable for the production of clothes? Let's start with the growing cycle. Hemp cultivators say the plant requires little fertilizer, can be grown just about anywhere, and doesn't need pesticides because it's naturally pest resistant. It can also be grown in the same soil for decades without the need for crop rotation because it replenishes the soil with nutrients. It also produces about twice as much fiber per acre as cotton and needs just a fraction of the water to grow. These are all factors that make hemp one of the most environmentally friendly crops grown on the planet.

Sellers say hemp is the most durable and yet softest of all the fabric crops, and it is warmer and more absorbent than cotton. It's naturally resistant to mold and mildew, and it shields and absorbs ultraviolet light better than other fabrics. Hemp fabric, which becomes softer with use, draws comparisons to linen. And hemp fibers don't weaken with repeated washings as synthetic fibers do.

Today, though hemp still isn't grown commercially on U.S. soil to produce clothing, you can find dozens of retailers that sell hemp garments that are made elsewhere. To shop for hemp online, check out these retailers:

- dankforest.com
- ecolution.com
- emperorshemp.com
- hempest.com
- hemphouse.com
- hempsisters.com
- hemptraders.com
- rawganique.com

How to Choose Safe Clothing

It's necessary to learn how to read clothing labels not just for what they say, but also for what they don't reveal to you. The identity of many chemicals used in synthetic clothing is considered proprietary company information. In addition, federal government regulations don't require that all chemicals used in synthetics be listed on labels. This section will explore ways that you as a consumer can make wise choices when buying clothes.

Tests You Can Use To Identify Fabrics

It's not always easy to distinguish between purely natural fabrics and blends of natural and synthetic fibers. If you want to determine whether a fabric is natural, synthetic, or a blend of the two, you can perform either a simple burn test or a household chemical test.

Depending on the temperature of the heat source, all fabric fibers will burn. But there are differences between natural fibers and synthetics in their burn rate and the various smells that are released. A burn test can help you to differentiate types of fabrics.

Exercise caution when doing this burn test. You will need to place water or soda in the bottom of a dish and have a lighter or match handy. Hold a small piece of fabric with tweezers and light it on fire. Most synthetics, because they are petroleum-based products, will melt and drip when burning.

The website www.fabrics.net features a series of tips on how to conduct these fabric identification tests and use the results to differentiate natural, synthetic, or blend fibers. Here is a summary of how the various fabrics react to heat:

Synthetic Fibers

Acetate – made from wood with many chemical additives, it cannot easily be extinguished when burning and leaves a hard ash similar to wood chips.

Acrylic – made from petroleum, it burns quickly with an acrid smell and leaves a soft ash.

Nylon – another petroleum product, it melts and smells like burning plastic.

Polyester – manufactured from petroleum and coal, it burns and melts simultaneously and leaves an ash that adheres to surfaces and produces a black smoke.

Rayon – almost pure cellulose, it ignites quickly, leaves little ash and smells like burning leaves.

Natural Fibers

Cotton – burns with a steady flame, emits a burning-leaf aroma, and leaves a very soft ash.

Linen – takes longer than cotton to ignite and leaves a brittle ash. Like cotton, it's easily extinguished.

Silk – this protein fiber burns easily, emits a smell like burning hair, and has an easily crumbled ash.

Wool – harder to ignite than silk, it also leaves a burning-hair smell, but the flame proves more difficult to keep steady.

You also can use two chemicals that are commonly found in the home or readily purchased in stores to distinguish between fiber types. Acetone is a nail polish remover ingredient that dissolves acetate while leaving other types of fibers undamaged. A liquid called Fiber-Etch, which is used in cutwork embroidery, dissolves cotton, linen, and other plant fibers. Using it to test a small fabric swatch can help you to determine if clothing is a blend and, if so, how much of a fabric is natural and how many of the fibers are synthetic.

Safe Cleaning and Storage of Clothes

Eco-friendly and human-health-friendly options are always available if you take the time to search for them and then use them once they are identified. Your choice of laundry detergents has environmental impacts that can actually be measured. The estimated carbon dioxide emission generated by an average load of laundry that is washed with conventional liquid laundry detergent is about 1.5 pounds; by contrast, carbon dioxide emission for laundry that is washed with conventional powdered detergent is about 1.8 pounds per load of clothes cleaned.

Seventh Generation is a Vermont-based company that offers eco-friendly and safe products, including natural fabric softeners and powdered and liquid laundry detergents. Company executives point out that if every household in the United States replaced just one 100-ounce bottle of petroleum-based liquid laundry detergent with Seventh Generation's 100-ounce bottle of vegetable-based detergent product, "we could save 460,000 barrels of oil, enough to heat and cool 27,000 U.S. homes for a year."

Tips for Eco- and Health-Friendly Cleaning

- If you buy a detergent, it should say "no fragrance" on the container. Even if the product says "unscented," it may still have a fragrance inside. A few products, such as Granny's Unscented Detergent, can be trusted, but you must do your homework to decipher which products are truly fragrance free.
- If you want a safe fragrance in your wash and on your clothes, consider adding an essential oil like rosemary. This can be a safe and effective alternative to synthetic chemical fragrances, but make sure you aren't allergic to essential oils before adding them.
- Use dryer balls instead of chemical fabric softeners. Dryer balls soften fabrics, eliminate static, and shorten drying time by up to 25 percent. Another eco-friendly alternative to chemical fabric softeners is to add a cup of ordinary household baking soda to the rinse cycle.

- To further diminish the environmental impact of cleaning your clothes, dry your laundry outside on a line instead of in a clothes dryer. Taking that step will cut your carbon footprint—the amount of carbon dioxide and other greenhouse gases you generate—by 4.4 pounds for every load of clothes you dry this way.
- To bleach clothes, try adding hydrogen peroxide to the wash. Another option is to soak the clothes overnight in eight parts of cold water to every one part of hydrogen peroxide, and then wash the clothes.

Tips for Silk Fabric Care

On the website www.wintersilks.com, the home page for the Winter-Silks Company based in Florida, you will find some helpful advice about how to care for your silk fabric clothing without resorting to abrasive or toxic chemicals. Here is a summary of their tips for silk care success:

Wash by hand. It may sound and feel old-fashioned, but washing silk by hand is an easy and safe way to keep the fabric looking new. Use a nonalkaline soap and lukewarm water. Any soap residue can be dissolved by adding pure white vinegar to the rinse water. Don't soak the silk for more than three or four minutes. Never use harsh detergents that contain bleach. And never wash in very hot or very cold water.

Machine wash. If you must wash your silk fabrics in a washing machine, use a nontoxic, biodegradable cleaning product. Silk Wash is one such product, made by WinterSilks, that works for both machine and hand washes. Use only lukewarm water in the machine.

Removing stains. Use only a nontoxic and biodegradable cleaning product and never use chlorine bleach. Spot Out is another WinterSilks cleaner that is effective. Remember that alcohol and soft drinks leave stains unless the fabric is treated quickly. Also remember that the alcohol in perfume and other personal care products can damage silk.

Fabric drying. For best results, dry your silk fabric naturally, but not in direct sunlight, as that fades the color and damages fibers. Gently squeeze the silk and roll it in a towel. Then lay it flat to dry. Shake the silk periodically to avoid stiffening. A warm iron—not a hot one—can be used to dry and press the fabric.

You Can Make Natural Clothing Dyes

If you want to avoid exposure to toxic commercial dyes in clothing and you're also feeling creative, making natural plant dyes may be a good option for you. Some of the plants that make good clothing dyes might even be found in your own backyard, as you will see from the list below. Others might be growing in the wild near your home. You will need to use blossoms in full bloom, and berries and nuts when they are mature and ripe.

For a detailed description of the steps you will need to take to prepare a dye bath for your clothing to soak in, go to www.pioneerthinking.com/naturaldyes.html. Here are examples of colors and some of the plants that provide the best dyes:

- orange: bloodroot, onion skin, carrot, and lilac
- brown: wild plum root, oak bark, dandelion root, and walnut hulls
- pink: strawberries, cherries, raspberries, and roses
- blue and purple: red cabbage, mulberries, blackberries, and hyacinth
- red: sumac, beets, chokecherries, and dried hibiscus flowers
- green: artichokes, spinach leaves, foxglove flowers, and black-eyed Susans
- yellow: turmeric, willow leaves, mimosa flowers, and hickory leaves

Natural Ways to Remove Pesky Stains

Rather than take risks with your health by applying or wearing toxic stain-resistant chemicals, why not try some safe old-fashioned methods that are proven to be effective? Some of the best advice for naturally removing stains from clothing can be found in *Betty's Book of Laundry Secrets* by Betty Faust and Maria Rodale. They recommend something very simple—using a scrub brush and a bar of mild soap that doesn't contain deodorants or chemical additives.

The key is to identify the stain before it is baked into the fabric by the drying process. That means spotting the smudge and taking action before you wash the clothing, or immediately afterward. Soak the spots in cold water, then vigorously rub the soap into the stain and rinse. If the stain is still there, repeat the process and soak the fabric for thirty minutes in cold water. This is when the scrub brush comes in handy. Without damaging the fabric, scrub the soap into the stain. As a last resort, gently blot the stain with a color-safe bleach. Use an oxygen bleach, not a chlorine bleach. Dilute with water, then rinse out the bleach.

Special stains require special attention. To remove mildew, for instance, wash the clothing in warm or hot water using oxygen bleach and line dry, preferably in direct sunlight. Sweat stains can also be removed by using sunlight's natural bleaching action. For oil or grease stains, apply baking soda or cornstarch to the affected area; put the cloth, stain side down, on a rag atop an ironing board; and iron the opposite side of the cloth.

Dry Your Clothes Courtesy of Nature

You can generate energy savings to support your financial health, and have much less negative impact on the health of the environment, if you simply allow Nature to dry and freshen your clothes for you. On the website www.planetgreen.com, you will find useful tips on how to dispense with you dryer and all of those fabric softeners and let the outdoor air do your work for you.

Use white vinegar in the rinse cycle to prevent the clothing from becoming stiff. Anywhere from one-half to three-quarters of a cup of vinegar in each wash load should keep the garments soft while drying.

Whether you are drying outdoors or inside a basement or on a porch, always use clothespins and clip the garments by their hemlines, though pinning T-shirts at the underarm also works well. Keep sufficient space between clothing items on the line to allow for faster drying. You can even create an all-natural linen spray for additional freshening power by consulting the Planet Green website www.planetg reen.com.

CHAPTER 7

The Dangerous Future of Clothing

Nanotechnology. Nanoparticles. Nanomaterials. Nanosilver. Nanotextiles. Not too long ago, neither those terms nor the products now connected to them would have held much meaning for most of us. We have rapidly entered a "brave new world" in the twenty-first century, where the manipulation of matter at the microscopic level affects even our selection of clothing.

What exactly are nanoparticles in nanotextiles produced by the new science of nanotechnology, and why is this mostly invisible layer of functionality appearing in so many name-brands of clothing? Is it a potential threat to the health of humans and the environment?

Let's start with a really simple definition of nanotechnology. It's the ability to manipulate molecules at a level smaller than the width of a human hair, down even to a level tinier than the human eye can see without a microscope. This manufacturing capability can result in a wide range of consumer products being made stronger, made more durable, and endowed with new qualities.

Silver in its nanosized form—usually reduced to be smaller in size than many viruses—is effective at killing microbes, which is why it now commonly appears in clothing to make the garments odor-resistant. It's also being marketed as a way to give clothes an antistain ability.

We are just now getting a glimpse at the potential long-term costs to human and environmental health of relying on silver nanoparticles in clothing to provide us with antistain and antibacterial agents. But since clothing manufacturers aren't required by law to disclose the presence of nanoparticles in the garments they produce and sell, we consumers are mostly uninformed about what we're putting on our skin.

Some clues about the presence of nanoparticles can be found in the terminology used by the clothing industry to market nanofabrics. Terms like "self-cleaning," "antibacterial," "antifungal," "stain repellant," and "static resistant," usually are indicators that nanoparticles have been embedded in the fibers.

Nanoparticles Release During Wash and Wear

Depending on the type of clothing and the presence of bleaching agents, washing nanotextiles can result in a substantial release of silver nanoparticles into the waterways of our natural environment through washing machine wastewater. That's the finding of a 2009 study published in the *Environmental Science &*

Technology journal (Geranio 2009). A team of Swiss scientists tested nine silver nanotextile articles of clothing by washing them and measuring the release of nanoparticles from their fibers.

When bleaching agents such as hydrogen peroxide or peracetic acid are used to wash the nanoclothing, the chemicals greatly accelerate the separation of nanoparticles from the fabric. There was also a big variation in the nanoparticles released based on the type of clothing and how the nanoparticles were embedded during manufacturing. Some clothing items released up to 45 percent of their total nanosilver content into wastewater.

An earlier study published in the same journal investigated the amount of silver released from nanosocks into wastewater and attempted to predict its fate in wastewater treatment plants. Arizona State University researchers tested six types of socks containing nanosilver and found some pairs leached as much as half of their nanosilver content into water, prompting the researchers to warn that "the high silver concentration may limit the disposal of the biosolids as agricultural fertilizer" once the nanosilver passes through wastewater treatment (Benn 2008).

Nanoparticles from clothing are also released during everyday wear. As the Swiss study team writes in their 2009 article, "A textile that is disposed at the end of its use phase has lost about 10 percent of its weight through abrasion during washing and usage, which suggests that particulate release may play a dominant role."

The first attempt to measure the release of silver nanoparticles from antibacterial fabrics as a result of human perspiration was documented in an April 2010 study in the journal, *Particle Fibre Toxicology.* Using a system of incubating the fabric in artificial sweat, researchers measured the amount of nanosilver released from clothing under conditions simulating everyday human wear. Releases in different clothing fabrics ranged up to 322 mg/kg of fabric weight, which is a lot. The quantity of silver released, which could have been absorbed by human skin if the clothing had been worn, was dependent on the fabric quality, the amount of silver coating, and the pH level of the sweat.

Based on the studies described above, we know that nanosilver in clothing can leach from the fabric under a variety of conditions—during washing and everyday wear—so the question now becomes, what potential risk is there to human and environmental health from our use of textiles containing nanoparticles?

12 Nanoclothing Examples (from among hundreds on the market)

260 Den Nanosilver Far Infrared Antiodor Healthy Socks

Manufacturer: Tsung-Hau Technology

Description: Nanosilver combined with fiber creates socks with antibacterial, disinfection, and deodorization qualities.

3XDry Essex Shirt

Manufacturer: Simms Fishing Products

Description: A silver-based nanofabric offers all-day sun protection, has an antiodor treatment "that lasts the lifetime of the garment," and repels moisture and "wicks perspiration away from the body."

4Season OG Pants

Manufacturer: Outlier

Description: A New York City product, its nanosphere coating is self-cleaning because the fabric's surface is coated in nanoscopic spikes that prevent stain molecules from bonding to fibers.

A La Mode Performance Long Sleeve Mock Neck

Manufacturer: Green Tee Apparel

Description: A fashionable long-sleeved top for golfing, it repels liquids, resists wrinkles, and has antimicrobial properties.

Agility Halter Dress

Manufacturer: Green Tee Apparel

Description: Designed for women golfers, the dress repels liquids, resists wrinkles, dries fast, and has antimicrobial features. A "100 percent poly pique nanotech" fabric.

Antibacterial Silver Athletic and Lounging Socks

Manufacturer: Sharper Image

Description: Sports socks knitted with cotton material that contains "millions of invisible silver nanoparticles" that are "naturally antibacterial and antifungal."

Smartcare and NANO-LEL Clothing

Manufacturer: Nordstrom Inc

Description: A "superior stain repellency" nanopants with "breathable comfort." It is made with a "Nano-Tex chemical process that binds the molecules of an industry-standard water repellent to the individual cotton fibers. This makes the fabric's water resistance more effective, more durable, and invisible to consumers."

Tencil Clothing

Manufacturer: Lenzing

Description: This is trumpeted as the first cellulose fiber to use a nanotechnology called Nanofibrils, which "optimize absorption of moisture with excellent cooling properties."

Steel Pants

Manufacturer: Beyond

Description: Made with something called Schoeller's Durable Dynamic with NanoSphere, these pants that convert to shorts have nanoparticles that make the garment "self-cleaning."

Nano-Tex Textiles

Manufacturer: Nano-Tex Inc.

Description: Its advertising says "a revolutionary technology" transforms the fabric in these garments at the nanolevel and "dramatically improves your favorite everyday clothing."

Resists Static Fabric

Manufacturer: Nano-Tex Inc.

Description: This clothing line "lets fabric repel lint, dust, and pet hair that normally clings to static attraction."

The Environmental Impact of Nanoparticle Release

As silver nanoparticles are leached from clothing and other consumer products and transit through the natural environment, they affect plant life by stunting its growth. That was the August 2010 finding of Duke University researchers who applied silver nanoparticles to outdoor fields of plants. They documented that the nanosilver reduced plant growth by 22 percent, and microbial biomass by 20 percent, compared to plant fields cultivated without nanosilver.

The scientists who presented these findings to the annual meeting of the Ecological Society of America (on August 4, 2010) noted that the nanoparticles released through wastewater end up at wastewater treatment plants, where they remain unaltered and accumulate in sludge. This sludge usually is trucked to crop fields where it's applied to soil as a fertilizer.

That process of toxic sludge dispersal may put portions of our nation's food supply at risk because the nanoparticles persist in the environment. They can affect plant growth, as the study determined, but also plant health because the plants depend on fungi and soil bacteria for nutrients. Both of these are significantly depleted by the antimicrobial nanoparticles.

"What we found was actually a little bit surprising," study coauthor Ben Colman told *Scientific American.* "We added lower concentrations of silver to a more complex system, but rather than find no measurable effect, we found that the silver nanoparticles significantly altered the plant growth, microbial biomass, and microbial activity."

More studies must be done to measure the effects of these nanoparticles on aquatic plants, insects, and fish. But the studies that have already been completed certainly raise enough troubling questions. A cautionary principle should be invoked in the use of nanoparticles in general, and in their use in clothing in particular.

In the January 31, 2010, issue of *Aquatic Toxicology,* a team of Danish researchers reported that silver nanoparticles "cause respiratory stress in Eurasian perch," apparently as a result of the particles interfering with fish gill function. In a similar fashion, a study by University of Florida scientists, published in a September 27, 2008, issue of *Environmental Toxicology & Chemistry,* determined that nanosilver and nanocopper "caused toxicity in all organisms tested," which included zebra fish, a plant species, and an algal species. Lethal concentrations were found at levels so low that the researchers admitted they were completely surprised by the finding.

Do Clothing Nanoparticles Endanger Human Health?

Though no studies have been conducted to determine the health dangers to humans of absorbing silver nanoparticles from clothing, at least not as of this writing, initial research has been done to assess how nanoparticles that have added to cosmetics, sunscreens, and personal care products might pose threats to human health. Nanoparticles are being added to skin products to force product ingredients to penetrate the body more rapidly and deeply, presumably making the products longer lasting and more effective. Up to two-thirds of sunblock and sunscreen products sold in the United States today now contain nanoparticles of titanium dioxide or zinc oxide, though few disclose this fact on the product labels. Out of the eight sunscreen products containing nanoparticles that were examined by *Consumer Reports* magazine in 2007, for example, only one disclosed their presence on the label.

Once nanoparticles penetrate the skin, they enter the bloodstream and gain free access to all of the major body organs, including passage through the blood-brain barrier. Numerous toxicology studies have warned that nanoparticles circulating through the human body may create unpredictable risks to health. For instance, an October 2005 study that was published in the journal *Toxicology In Vitro* found that silver nanoparticles had toxic effects on the liver cells of lab animals, subjecting the cells to oxidative stress.

As a November 22, 2007, article in *The Economist* noted, "Research on animals suggests that nanoparticles can even evade some of the body's natural defense systems and accumulate in the brain, cells, blood, and nerves. Studies show there is the potential for such materials to reach the lungs and cause inflammation; to move from the lungs to other organs; to have surprising biological toxicity; to move from within the skin to the lymphatic system; and possibly to move across cell membranes."

Clothing manufacturers that are now trumpeting nanoparticles technology to consumers, like the cosmetics and personal care industries before them, make many unfounded assumptions about health and safety based on insufficient research data. A June 2006 commentary in *Nature* spotlighted this trend by noting how "the chemicals industry has blithely assumed that if large grains are safe, smaller ones (nanoparticles) will be too. But that assumption is coming under increasing scrutiny and is not necessarily always valid."

Subsequent to publication of the *Nature* article, three studies appeared and cast even more doubt about the safety of silver nanoparticles:

1. "The potential side effects of these nanoparticles (silver) have not been studied thoroughly yet," commented the authors of a May 27, 2010, study in the journal *Immunopharmacology & Immunotoxicology.* So the team of researchers examined the toxic effects of silver nanoparticles on macrophages, one of the body's most important immune cells. They found that exposure of the cells to the nanoparticles resulted in "a significant decrease in cell viability" at a dosage of 1 part per million up to 25 parts per million of nanoconcentrations, which also produced a "considerable decline" in nitric oxide production by the macrophages.
2. To measure the effect of silver nanoparticles on coronary cells and the aortic heart rings of lab animals, scientists writing in a December 15, 2009, issue of *Toxicology Letters* said they discovered that the particles affected cells in several different ways, both with high and low concentrations that either increased cell proliferation or inhibited proliferation. These biological effects were observed based on particle size could have unpredictable effects on the human heart.
3. "Despite the widespread use of nanosilver, there is a serious lack of information concerning the biological activities of nanosilver on human tissue

cells," observed a German team of researchers writing in a May 2009 issue of *Langenbecks, Archives of Surgery.* They tested the effects of silver nanoparticles on human stem cells and found that at high concentrations, these particles had cytotoxic effects (cytotoxic refers to any agent or process that kills cells.)

Silver nanoparticles in clothing may ultimately be found to have effects on the human body similar to the adverse health impacts documented from inhaling ultrafine particles of a similar size, mostly produced by vehicle emissions and absorbed from the atmosphere. No less a source than the *Journal of Nanoscience & Nanotechnology,* in an August 9, 2009, article titled "Nanoparticles and the brain: cause for concern?" pointed out that both nanoparticles and ultrafine particles may be neurotoxins with unpredictable effects on the brain and central nervous system.

"More studies are needed to test the hypothesis that inhaled nanoparticles cause neurodegenerative effects," wrote the University of Rochester scientists. "Some but probably not the majority of nanoparticles will have a significant toxicity (hazard) potential, and this will pose a significant risk if there is a sufficient exposure."

The Worst Futuristic Clothing Idea Ever!

Imagine being able to spray chemical clothing from a can directly onto your skin in whatever style or design that you choose. This is not or science fiction. It's science reality, and the invention will appear in 2011 as a consumer product called Fabrican, which is marketed out of Britain.

Scientists at Imperial College in London developed a liquid clothing spray made of cotton fibers, polyester, plastics, and solvents that harden on contact with the skin to form a reusable garment that is washable. All you need to do is peel it off for re-use, or to be discarded, depending on your fashion whim.

This is how the www.fabricanltd.com website describes its product: "The technology opens new vistas for personalized fashion, allowing individual touches to be added to manufactured garments, or even impromptu alterations. Garments could incorporate fragrances, active substances, or conductive materials to interface with information technology."

While the use of this chemical mixture of solvents, polyesters, and plastics might make sense for use as spray-on bandages, which could be applied directly to a wound without adding pressure, its use as a second skin for the entire body raises many troubling health questions. There is no indication on the product website that these combinations of chemicals—many of the solvents, for instance, are toxic—have ever been tested for the short-term, much less long-term, impacts on human health. To incorporate additional fragrances and other active substances into the chemical mixture, as the manufacturer proposes, only further complicates the health uncertainties.

Organic Fibers Create a More Planet-Friendly Future

When it comes to ensuring the future health of the environment, there is no comparison between natural and synthetic fibers. Natural organic fibers grow as a result of energy that is directly generated by the sun, whose rays are our planet's most abundant renewable resource. Once their usefulness ends, these natural fibers biodegrade and readily integrate back into the ecosystem.

Synthetic fibers mostly come from a nonrenewable resource—fossil fuels—and they rarely biodegrade, at least not in our lifetimes. With the introduction of nanosilver particles, fibers can last even longer, becoming virtually indestructible.

What we choose to put on our bodies, whether it's clothes, or cosmetics and personal care products, affects the health of our outer natural environment just as severely as it does the health of our inner bodily environment. As this book has demonstrated, conventional processes for manufacturing synthetic fibers generate more types of chemical contaminants and environmental degradation than you might have previously imagined.

Though the fabrics manufacturing industry hasn't been very forthcoming with data about its use and release of chemicals into the environment, the study of industry practices done in 2005 by the Greenpeace Research Laboratories in Britain, discussed in Chapter 2, uncovered enough information to create a disturbing profile. Here is a recap of the eleven most severe pollution problems from textile manufacturing that these scientists, and other researchers in separate studies, have identified:

- A solvent used to clean wool, trichloroethylene, is a cancer-causing chemical, possibly at any exposure level, and seeps into ecosystems during the manufacturing process.
- During fabric bleaching, a hormone disruptive chemical called EDTA is often used, and it persists in the effluent released by manufacturing plants, which means it can bioaccumulate in the environment.
- Optical brightener detergents also persist in ecosystems after textile plants release wastewater effluent.
- A whole class of synthetic dyes, especially Direct dyes using formaldehyde, has proven toxic to aquatic systems. Chrome dyes bioaccumulate in many aquatic species and are toxic.

- Phthalates bind dyes to fabric, but some of these plasticizers are toxic to both human and animal life. One of them, DEHP, is a proven reproductive toxin.
- Formaldehyde is released into the environment from wrinkle-free and shrinkage-free garments, posing risks to both human and aquatic life.
- Flame retardants are now found everywhere in the environment, and though textiles account for less than half of the toxic levels, they still contribute unnecessarily to the problem.
- Triclosan, an antibacterial and antifungicidal finish, leaches from clothes in the wash and from textile plants through wastewater to bioaccumulate in ecosystems as a toxin.
- Textile mills typically release wastewater that contains toxic heavy metals, such as zirconium and cobalt, from fabric dyes.
- Now that the insecticide permethrin is being added to clothing during the manufacturing process, its residue is being channeled through wastewater into the environment, where it's toxic to plant and animal life.
- Increasing levels of nanosilver are being released and contribute to the toxic brew accumulating in ecosystems.

"Effluents and sludge from production processes cannot be safely deposited into ecosystems," note the authors of the book about sustainability practices, *Cradle to Cradle,* "so they are often buried or burned as hazardous waste. The fabric itself is sold all over the world, used, then thrown 'away'—which usually means it is either incinerated, releasing toxins, or placed in a landfill. Even in the rather short life span of the fabric, its particles have abraded into the air and been taken into people's lungs."

Greenpeace laboratory researchers summarized their findings about the chemicals used in manufacturing clothes using this language: "The textile industry and its products give rise to a wide range of environmental and toxicological impacts. However, due to the complexity and range of chemistry involved and the lack of available data, an accurate assessment of this impact is difficult. Efforts have been made in Europe, at least, to avoid chemicals of high concern; unfortunately, this cannot be taken for granted worldwide."

The report might have added that since most clothing sold in the world originates in countries outside of Europe, "chemicals of high concern" are found everywhere. The European tendency to limit toxic risks is a public policy that is not yet on display in the United States, which remains one of the largest consumer markets for foreign-manufactured synthetic, nonorganic, and nanotech fibers.

Finding Our Way Back

Here and there we can see a few positive clothing trends afoot. One example is the emergence of soy and bamboo fibers and a vegetable fiber called saluyot. These new natural forms of textiles are being created without any reliance on petrochemicals or nanotechnology. They are safe for both humans and the environment.

But how many consumers know about these new natural clothing fibers? Had you ever wondered what happens to your items of clothing when you discard them? Did you think they go to a landfill and quickly degrade harmlessly back into the environment?

If you're like most people, you probably never gave these sorts of questions a passing consideration. Out of sight, out of mind! Yet, future generations will be forced to live with our environmental mistakes unless we ask the right questions and come up with the right answers.

If this book accomplishes anything worthwhile, we hope it's the heightening of awareness that synthetic clothing can put not only human health at risk, but environmental health as well. It's an interconnected web, and every individual decision that we make contributes to either strengthening or weakening that web of life.

Now that you are aware that synthetic clothing doesn't biodegrade like natural fibers and that these synthetics will be a disposal headache for many generations to come, you can make a personal contribution to the solution. It's a process that starts with holding ourselves and each other accountable for purchasing and using only safe natural products that are designed to keep us and our planet healthy.

Using natural fibers whenever possible is a long-term investment in our personal health, in the health of our children, and just as importantly, in the health of our planet. Clothes shouldn't be ecological time bombs. They should be expressions of our desire to live in harmony with our bodies and with the Garden of Eden that is planet Earth, which we were blessed to be born into.

Appendix

Companies That Produce Safe Clothing

Dozens of manufacturers now produce safe, natural, organic clothing. For example, Near Sea Naturals makes yarns from plant-based fibers and Janice's makes natural clothing for people with chemical sensitivities. You will also find companies listed here that make chemical-free cloth diapers and other products for babies and young children.

(Note: The following information was accurate as of July 2010.)

Baby Clothes

BabyNaturopathics.com —An entire line of certified organic cotton infant clothing can be found here, including bibs, shirts, pants, hats, and kimonos.

Babyworks.com —This Oregon family business carries organic cotton baby clothes of all types, along with nontoxic diaper products.

Hanna Andersson Baby Clothes (www.hannaandersson.com) —Children's clothes produced by this company have been certified by the Okeo-Tex Standard 100 as being free of more than one hundred harmful substances. Only environmentally responsible dyes are used in organic cotton clothes for every member of the family.

Hatley Baby Clothes (hatleystore.com) —No azo dyes are used in these organic cotton products and only nonchlorinated bleach is used on the fabrics.

Organic Adobe Baby Clothes (www.organicadobe.com) —These organic cotton clothes use nontoxic dyes and are guaranteed to be free of formaldehyde, flame retardants, and other toxins that are commonly mainstream baby products. The company was founded in Santa Cruz, California.

Organicgrace.com —Nontoxic options for healthy living is the motto of this company in Garberville, California, which sells organic cotton and wool baby products, and hemp and organic cotton "moon pads" for women's menstrual cycles.

Preciousdignity.com —Quality cloth diapers made of eco-friendly fabrics are a specialty; every item is made in Columbus, Ohio.

Speesess Baby Clothes (www.speesees.com) —These organic cotton baby clothes use environmentally sound herbal dyes.

Clothes for All Ages

Ecowise.com —Opened in Austin, Texas, in 1990, this "earth-friendly everything store" carries an organic line of clothing that includes men's and women's apparel in hemp and cotton.

Fairindigo.com —This company in Madison, Wisconsin, features eco-friendly fashions, an organic line of clothing, and a "fair trade" attitude toward suppliers who pay their employees fair wages.

Greenfibres.com —Not only does this British company carry organic clothing for men, women, and children, it also sells Sonett eco-clothes and cleaning products that use organic ingredients.

Janices.com —Janice is a real person in North America who created a natural organic clothing line for people with chemical sensitivities.

Nearseanaturals.com —Based in New Mexico, this company is a member of the Organic Trade Association and features knit and woven fabrics, and yarns made from organic plant-based fibers.

Organic-cotton-co.com —Founded by Jon Cloud, an organic food and fiber activist in Toronto, Canada, the company philosophy is "organic products heal the Earth." The certified organic pima cotton product line consists of underwear for women, men, and children; socks for babies to adults; bras; T-shirts; hoodies; and long-sleeve undershirts.

OrganicWearUSA.com —This company offers baby clothes without bleach or petroleum-based dyes or inks, and fibers grown without pesticides and insecticides.

Patagonia.com —This company based in California uses only organic cotton in its clothing for men and women, and specializes in outdoor wear.

Roguenaturalliving.com —This Oregon-based company features "nontoxic goods for the New Green

Revolution" and sells organic clothing for youth, women (lingerie is one item), men, and unisex.

Rootedtonature.com —This online store specializes in natural fiber clothing made from organic cotton, wool, hemp, silk, and even soy and bamboo fibers.

Wintersilks.com —Based in Jacksonville, Florida, this company sells thirty-two different types of silk fabrics and clothing, including herringbone for shirts, pants and blazers, silk cashmere, silk linen, and other blends with angora and bamboo.

Organic Cotton Clothing Providers (ask for these brands at clothing stores)

Recycleatee—Organic clothing for the eco-friendly.

Faerie's Dance—Women's fashions in organic cotton, hemp, tencel, and soy.

The Oko Box—The latest styles in organic cotton, hemp, bamboo, tencel, and soy.

Live Life Organics—Organic clothing, plantable hangtags, and water-based inks.

Onno Textiles—Organic cotton, bamboo, and hemp T-shirts.

Kasper Organics—Organic cotton clothing, and hemp clothing.

Baby Naturopathics Inc—Embroidered organic baby clothing.

Butterfly Maidens—Unbleached and naturally dyed organic clothing for women and children.

Cultivate Kids—Organic infant and toddler T-shirts.

VivaLocaWear—Organic T-shirts for students and activists.

Shanghai Fashionorganic—Organic clothing and fabric from China, made from bamboo, organic cotton, hemp, and soybeans.

Kook Wear—Environmentally friendly clothing for action sports enthusiasts.

Nubius Organics—Apparel, toys, and accessories for babies and kids.

Go Natural Baby—Organic cotton baby and children's clothes.

Maternity Jeans—Organic cotton maternity jeans and clothes.

Tees 4 Trees—Earth-friendly apparel that celebrates nature.

Organic by Nature—Affordable organic children's clothing.

Byrnt Organics—All-organic vintage surf-inspired men's and women's denim and knits.

Essere Organics—The finest natural, eco-friendly, and organic products.

Organic Baby Clothing—Boutique-quality organic baby clothes.

Jute and Jackfruit—Handmade, designer organic cotton women's dresses, tops, and jackets.

A Consumer's Resource Guide

You will find listed here groups and organizations that promote safe clothing options or do consumer research on clothing. These include the La Leche League International, which offers advice and support to women who breast-feed, and websites that provide useful suggestions to women who choose to go bra free for health or other reasons.

About Organic Cotton (aboutorganiccotton.org)

This group keeps a list of companies that cultivate and sell organic cotton.

La Leche League International (www.llli.org)

A breast-feeding advocacy group that is a great resource for mothers and mothers-to-be.

Organic Consumers Association (www.organicconsumers.org)

Represents about 850,000 people and businesses dedicated to promoting and protecting natural foods and organic products.

Organic Exchange (www.organicexchange.org)

These clothing companies are committed to expanding organic agriculture and the use of organically grown fibers.

Organic Trade Association (www.ota.com)

This business association promotes trade in organic products and maintains a list of 1,600 companies that sell or manufacture organic products.

Clothing Chemicals to Avoid

The European Union and independent chemists and labs in Europe have compiled an extensive list of all chemicals that are used in clothing and pose a potential threat to human and wildlife health. The following list gives you, the consumer, information that will help you to identify these chemicals so you can avoid them whenever you encounter their names in association with clothing manufacturing practices.

Note: The Norwegian Textile Panel's list of hazardous chemicals can be found at http://www.greennow.net/Tekstiler/Chemicals.htm.

Pretreatment of Clothing

Alkylphenol ethoxylates: Used as surfactants in detergents during the production process, these hormone-disruptive chemicals persist in nature and can be toxic to aquatic life.

Nonylphenol and nonylphenol ethoxylates: Recommended that these substances never be applied in the production of textiles and that a maximum limit for unintentional contamination not exceed 30ppm.

Octylphenol and octylphenol ethoxylates: Banned in Norway for use in clothing.

Alpha.-sulfo-.omega.-(nonylphenoxy)-poly(oxy-1, 2 ethanediyl, ammonium salt: Recommended that these substances never be used in textiles and that unintentional contamination of finished products not exceed 30ppm.

Other alkylphenol ethoxylates: Should not be applied in the production of textiles and unintentional contamination should not exceed 30ppm.

Organic Solvents

1, 1, 1, 2-Tetrachloroethane: Should never be used.

1, 1, 2, 2-Tetrachloroethane: Should never be used.

Pentachloroethane: Should never be used.

Benzene: Used in textile dyeing, but should not be.

Carbon tetrachloride: Banned in Norway due to ozone depletion effect.

Toluene: Should never be used.

N, N-Dimethylformamide: Should never be used.

1, 1-Oxybis-2-propanol: A textile bleach that should never be used.

Textile Dyeing

Azo dyes: These 25 dyes are banned because they release the carcinogen arylamines. (For the complete list refer to the website listed in section entitled "Clothing Chemicals to Avoid".)

Disperse dyes: These 22 dyes ranging from Disperse Blue 1 to Disperse Brown 1 are used to dye synthetic fibers, may cause cancer or allergies, and should never be used. (For the complete list refer to the website listed in section entitled "Pretreatment of Clothing".)

Acid dyes: These 7 dyes may cause cancer or allergies and should never be used. (For the complete list refer to the website listed in section entitled "Pretreatment of Clothing".)

Basic dyes: Basic Red 9 and Basic Violet 14 are Cationic dyes that may cause cancer and should never be used in any process.

Direct dyes: These 4 substantive dyes—Direct Black 38, Direct Blue 6, Direct Red 28, and Direct Blue

1—may cause cancer or allergies and should never be used.

Textile Finishing Treatments

Formaldehyde: Used to make textiles shrinkage resistant and wrinkle resistant, and as a binding agent for ink, it is a carcinogen and an allergen. Norway recommends the use of formaldehyde-free resins.

Metals and metal Ranging compounds: from mercury to copper, they are used in a variety of ways in the processing of synthetic fibers. Various prohibitions and limitations apply to their use in Norway. (For the complete list refer to the website listed in section entitled "Pretreatment of Clothing".)

Organotin compounds: Used as catalysts in the production of synthetic fibers and to prevent the smell of sweat in clothing, 14 of these compounds are either banned outright in Norway or their use is limited. They have shown hormone disruptive properties even at low concentrations. (For the complete list refer to the website listed in section entitled "Pretreatment of Clothing".)

Flame retardants: Not recommended for clothes sold or produced in Norway because "it is possible to reduce flammability of clothes and textiles in other ways than by applying chemical flame retardants.".

Brominated flame retardants: Nine are listed as banned or limitations are place on their use in Norway. They are persistent in the environment and bioaccumulative in humans and wildlife. (For the complete list refer to the website listed in section entitled "Pretreatment of Clothing".)

Other flame retardants: Six other types of retardants are either banned or limited in Norwegian textiles. (For the complete list refer to the website listed in section entitled "Pretreatment of Clothing".)

Organochlorines: These solvents include triclosan, which is used to prevent bacterial growth in clothing. Most are either banned in Norway or their use is restricted.

Chlorinated benzenes, toluenes, etc.: Thirteen of these solvents are listed and warnings issued about their use, especially because safer alternatives exist. (For the complete list refer to the website listed in section entitled "Pretreatment of Clothing".)

Chlorinated phenols: These fungicides and pesticides can cause serious health damage to humans and environmental damage. (For the complete list refer to the website listed in section entitled "Pretreatment of Clothing".)

Phthalates: Used as plasticizers in fabrics, eight of them are either banned or restricted in Norway. (For the complete list refer to the website listed in section entitled "Pretreatment of Clothing".)

Asbestos: Fibers coated in asbestos are still used in some countries. Norway bans the use of six of the most common.

Pesticides: Mostly used in the cultivation of natural fibers, 24 are listed by Norway as either being banned or restricted. (For the complete list refer to the website listed in section entitled "Pretreatment of Clothing".)

References

Chapter 1

"Acrylics linked to breast cancer." *Sydney Morning Herald,* April 5, 2010.

Ashizawa, K. et al. Breast Form Changes Resulting From a Certain Brassiere. *Journal of Human Ergol* (Tokyo). June 1990;19:53–62.

Becher, H. et al. Reproductive factors and familial predisposition for breast cancer by age 50 years. A case-control family study for assessing main effects and possible gene-environment interaction. *International Journal of Epidemiology.* February 2003;32:38–48.

Bellis, Mary. "The History of Panty Hose." Inventors.about.com.

Bellis, Mary. "The History of Nylon and Neoprene." Inventors.about.com.

Beral, V. et al. Breast cancer and breast-feeding: collaborative reanalysis of individual data from 47 epidemiological studies in 30 countries. *Lancet.* July 20, 2002;360:187–95.

Clarke, CA. et al. Population attributable risk of breast cancer in white women associated with immediately modifiable risk factors. *BMC Cancer.* June 27, 2006;6:170.

Cone, Marla. "Testing Finds Traces of Carcinogen in Bath Products." *Los Angeles Times,* February 9, 2007.

Darbre, PD. et al. Concentrations of Parabens in Human Breast Tumors. *Journal of Applied Toxicology.* 2004;24:5–13.

Darbre, PD. et al. Metalloestrogens: An Emerging Class of Inorganic Xenoestrogens with Potential to Add to the Oestrogenic Burden of the Human Breast. *Journal of Applied Toxicology.* 2006;26:191–7.

De Kretser, DM. Are sperm counts really falling? *Reproductive Fertility Dev.* 1998;10:93–5.

Dixon, JM. et al. Risk of breast cancer in women with palpable breast cysts: a prospective study. *Lancet.* May 22, 1999;353:1742–5.

"Do bras cause breast cancer?" www.BraFree.o rg.

"Do bras cause fibrocystic disease?" www.BraFr ee.org.

Elegbe, IA, and Elegbe I. Quantitiative relationships of *Candida albicans* infections and dressing patterns in Nigerian women. *American Journal of Public Health.* April 1983;4:450–2.

Epstein, Samuel MD. *Toxic Beauty.* Dallas: BenBella Books, 2009.

Fisher, AA. Unique reactions of scrotal skin to topical agents. *Cutis.* December 1989;44:445–7.

Hsieh, CC, and Trichopoulos, D. Premenopausal women who do not wear bras had half the risk of breast cancer compared to bra users. *European Journal Cancer.* 1991;27:131–5.

Kett, K. et al. Axillary lymph drainage as a prognostic factor of survival in breast cancer. *Lymphology.* December 2002;35:161–70.

Kunzelman, Michael. "Women say Victoria's Secret bras cause rashes." Associated Press, April 9, 2009.

Labreche, F., and Goldberg, MS. et al. Postmenopausal breast cancer and occupational exposures. *Occupational Environmental Medicine.* April 2010;67:263–9.

Lee, YA. et al. The effects of skin pressure by clothing on circadian rhythms of core temperature and salivary melatonin. *Chronobiol Int.* November 2000;17:783–93.

Marples, Gareth. "The History of the Bra—An Uplifting Story." Sept. 10, 2008. TheHistoryOf.net.

Miyatsuji, A. et al. Effects of clothing pressure caused by different types of brassieres on autonomic nervous system activity evaluated by heart rate variability power spectral analysis. *Journal Physiol Anthropol Appl Human Sci.* January 2002;21:67–74.

Nussdorf, Maggie Rollo, and Nussdorf, Stephen B. *Dress for Health: The New Clothes-Consciousness.* Harrisburg, Pa.: Stackpole Books, 1980.

Poole, Oliver. "British Study Links Bras to Cysts and Breast Cancer." *Sunday Telegraph,* Oct. 31, 2000.

Shockney, Lillie. "Are Breast Cancer Rates Really Going Down?" Yahoo Health, Jan. 10, 2007. http:/

/health.yahoo.com/experts/breastcancer/2500/are-breast-cancer-rates.

Shockney, Lillie. "Does Your Bra Fit Correctly?" Yahoo Health, Sept. 11, 2008. http://health.yahoo.com/experts/breastcancer/5872/does-your-bra-fit.

Shockney, Lillie. "Ill-Fitting Bras and Breast Cancer." Yahoo Health, Dec. 18, 2008. http://health.yahoo.com/experts/breastcancer/6271/ill-fitting-bras-and.

Singer, Sydney Ross, and Grismaijer, Soma. *Dressed to Kill: The Link Between Breast Cancer and Bras.* Garden City Park, New York: Avery Publishing Group, 1995.

"Stiletto warning for pregnant women." BBC News, June 15, 2010.

Tiemessen, CH, Evers, JL, and Bots, RS. Tight-fitting underwear and sperm quality. *Lancet.* June 29, 1996;347:1844–5.

Vaughan, Elizabeth R. www.vaughanintegrative.com.

Walsh, John. "A Social History of the Bra." *Independent UK,* August 29, 2007. http://www.alternet.org/story/59877/.

Weiss, Marisa MD. "10 Breast Cancer Myths Debunked." *Prevention,* Dec. 4, 2006.

White, RS. et al. Environmentally Persistent Alkylphenolic Compounds Are Estrogenic. *Endocrinology.* 1994;135:175–82.

Willingham, Val. "Flip-flops aren't always easy on the feet." CNN News, August 6, 2010.

"Women risk feet in fashion's name." BBC News, September 7, 2009.

Zeng, T. et al. Long-term Breast-feeding Lowers Mother's Breast Cancer Risk. *American Journal Epidemiology.* 2001;152:1129–1135.

Chapter 2

"An Overview of Textiles Processing and Related Environmental Concerns." Greenpeace Research Laboratories, University of Exeter UK, June 2005.

Blum, A, Gold, MD, and Ames, BN. Children Absorb Tris-BP Flame Retardant from Sleepwear: Urine Contains the Mutagenic Metabolite, 2,3-Dibromopropanol. *Science.* September 15, 1978;201:1020–23.

Brookstein, David. "Health effects of formaldehyde in textiles." Institute of Textile and Apparel Product Safety in testimony before the U.S. Senate Subcommittee on Consumer Protection, Product Safety and Insurance, April 28, 2009.

Burke, Kelly. "Chinese Textiles could pose cancer risk." *Sydney Morning Herald,* May 21, 2007.

"CPSC Bans Tris-Treated Children's Garments." U.S. Consumer Product Safety Commission, April 7, 1977 (Release # 77-030.)

Darnerud, PO. Toxic effects of brominated flame retardants in man and in wildlife. *Environ Int.* September 2003;29:841–53.

Donovan, J, and Skotnicki-Grant, S. Allergic contact dermatitis from formaldehyde textile resins in surgical uniforms and nonwoven textile masks. *Dermatitis.* March 2007;18:40–4.

Etzel, Ruth A. "Formaldehyde in Textiles and Consumer Products." Testimony on behalf of the American Academy of Pediatrics before the U.S. Commerce, Science and Transportation Subcommittee on Consumer Protection, Product Safety, and Insurance, April 28, 2009.

"Evaluation of Alleged Unacceptable Formaldehyde Levels in Clothing." Ministry of Consumer Affairs, Government of New Zealand, updated 07-05-2008, http://www.consumeraffairs.govt.nz/policylawresearch/product-safety.

"Fabric Identification Burn Test." http://www.fabrics.net/fabricsr.asp.

"Final Clarification of Statement of Policy: Standard for the Flammability of Children's Sleepwear." Federal Register, January 19, 1999, vol.64, no.11:2832–2833.

"Formaldehyde allergy." DermNet New Zealand, http://dermnetnz.org/dermatitis/formaldehype-allergy.html.

Fowler, JF. Formaldehyde as a textile allergen. *Current Problems Dermatology.* 2003;31:156–65.

Fowler, JF. et. al. Allergic contact dermatitis from formaldehyde resins in permanent press clothing: an underdiagnosed cause of generalized dermatitis. *Journal American Academy of Dermatology.* December 1992;27:962–8.

Gold, MD, Blum, A, and Ames, BN. Another flame retardant, tris-(1,3-dichloro-2-propyl)-phosphate, and its expected metabolites are mutagens. *Science.* May 19, 1978;200:785–7.

"Lessen Your Baby's Toxic Load: Clothing." Environmental Working Group, November 13, 2008, http://www.ewg.org/node/27359.

Masahiko, I. et al. Changes of Free Formaldehyde Quantity in Non-Iron Shirts by Washing and Storage. *Journal of Health Science.* 1999;45:412–17.

"Natural Baby, Poisonous World." Environmental Working Group, May 16, 2007, http://www.ewg.org/node/21581.

Pratt, Andy. "Science Outreach: Formaldehyde." University of Canterbury, New Zealand, http://www.outreach.canterbury.ac.nz/podcasts/formaldehyde.shtml. (Accessed May 27, 2009.)

Rao, Sanath. et al. Detection of formaldehype in textiles by chromotropic acid method. *Indian Journal of Dermatology.* November 1, 2004.

"Regulations for Textile and Clothing Products." U.S. Consumer Product Safety Commission, http://www.cpsc.gov/Trans/textiles.html, March 2009.

Rodriguez, Robert. "California Farmers Provide Clothing Retailers with Organic Cotton." *Knight Ridder/Tribune Business News,* May 9, 1999.

The Fire Retardant Dilemma. *Science.* October 12, 2007;318.

U.S. Consumer Product Safety Commission National Burn Center Reporting System, Division of Hazard Analysis, September 2004.

Chapter 3

"An Overview of Textiles Processing and Related Environmental Concerns." Greenpeace Research Laboratories, University of Exeter UK, June 2005.

Arisu, K. et al. Tinuvin P in a spandex tape as a cause of clothing dermatitis. *Contact Dermatitis.* May 1992;26:311–6.

"Disperse Blue 1: CAS No.2475-45-8." Report on Carcinogens, Eleventh Edition. www.niehs.NIH.gov.

"Dyes and Chemical Sensitivities." Lotus Organics. www.lotusorganics.com.

"Electrostatic Discharge." http://www.geocities.com/emsafety/electrostatic_discharge.htm.

Fitzgerald, Randall. *The Hundred Year Lie: How to Protect Yourself from the Chemicals That Are Destroying Your Health.* New York: Plume/Penguin, 2007.

Garcia, Ana, and Mamoun, Fred. "Lawsuit Talk Over Baby Clothes, Parents claim Carter's clothing causes rash." NBC Los Angeles, November 12, 2008.

Grimshaw, Vicki. "The Skin Friendly Home, From Sofas to Synthetic Clothes, a guide to reducing your family's skin problems." *Daily Mail* (London), May 21, 2002.

Haines, Lester. "30,000 volt synthetic jacket menaces OZ." *The Register,* September 16, 2005, http://www.theregister.uk/2005/09/16/static_jacket/print.html.

Hatch, KL, and Maibach, HI. Textile dye dermatitis. *Journal American Academy of Dermatology.* April 1995;32:631–9.

"Household chemicals may be linked to infertility." UCLA School of Public Health, January 30, 2009.

Jancin, Bruce. "Suspect textile contact dermatitis? Think blue: synthetic dyes are the big culprits." *Skin and Allergy News,* International Medical News Group, 2004.

Khanna, M, and Sasseville, D. Occupational contact dermatitis to textile dyes in airline personnel. *American Journal of Contact Dermat.* December 2001;12:208–10.

Lazarov, A. et al. Atypical and unusual clinical manifestations of contact dermatitis to clothing (textile contact dermatitis): case presentation and review of the literature. *Dermatology Online Journal.* August 2003;9:1.

Lazarov, A. Textile dermatitis in patients with contact sensitization in Israel: a 4-year prospective study. *Journal European Acad Dermatol Venerol.* September 2004;18:531–7.

Pratt, M, and Taraska, V. Disperse blue dyes 106 and 124 are common causes of textile dermatitis and should serve as screening allergens for this condition. *American Journal Contact Dermat.* March 2000;11:30–41.

Ricci, G. et al. Use of textiles in atopic dermatitis: care of atopic dermatitis. *Current Problems Dermatology.* 2006;33:127–43.

Shafik, A. Effect of different types of textile fabric on spermatogenesis: an experimental study. *Urology Res.* 1993;21:367–70.

Shafik, A. et al. Effect of different types of textile fabric on spermatogenesis: electrostatic potentials generated on the surface of the human scrotum by wearing different types of fabric. *Archives of Androl.* Sep–Oct. 1992;29:147–50.

Shafik, A. Effect of different types of textiles on male sexual activity. *Archives of Androl.* Sep–Oct. 1996;37:111–5.

"Stain repellent chemical linked to thyroid disease in adults." The Peninsula College of Medicine and Dentistry, January 21, 2010. www.pms.ac.uk.

"Toxic Cancer-Causing Dyes Found in China Garments." *Daijiworld* (India), July 31, 2010. www.daijiworld.com.

Warshall, Peter. "Inventory of Synthetic Fibers." *Whole Earth,* Summer 1997.

Wolf, R. Et. al. Contact dermatitis in military personnel. *Clinical Dermatology.* Jul–Aug 2002;20:439–44.

Zimniewska, M. et al. The Influence of Clothes Made from Natural and Synthetic Fibres on the Activity of the Motor Units in Selected Muscles in the Forearm—Preliminary Studies. *Fibres and Textiles in Eastern Europe.* October–December 2002:55–59.

Chapter 4

Abdel-Rahman, A. et al. Neurological deficits inducted by malathion, DEET, and permethrin, alone or in combination in adult rats. *Journal Toxicology Environmental Health A.* February 27, 2004;67:331–56.

Abdel-Rahman, A, Shetty, AK, and Abou-Donia, MB. Subchronic dermal application of N, N-diethyl m-toluamide (DEET) and permethrin to adult rats, alone or in combination, causes diffuse neuronal cell death and cytoskeletal abnormalities in the cerebral cortex and the hippocampus, and Purkinje neuron loss in the cerebellum. *Exp Neurol.* November 2001;172:153–71.

Abou-Donia, MB. et al. Co-exposure to pyrdiostigmine bromide, DEET, and/or permethrin causes sensorimotor deficit and alterations in brain acetycholinesterase activity. *Pharmacol Biochem Behav.* February 2004;77:253–62.

Appel, KE. et al. Risk assessment of Bundeswehr (German Federal Armed Forces) permethrin-impregnated battle dress uniforms(BDU). *Int J Hyg Environ Health.* March 2008;211:88–104.

Barr, DB. et al. Urinary concentrations of metabolites of pyrethroid insecticides in the general U.S. population: national health and nutrition examination survey 1999–2002. *Environ Health Perspect.* June 2010;118:742–8.

Brinkley, Mark. "The Corps in Iraq bans synthetic clothing off-base over the risk of burns." Leathernec k.com, April 18, 2006.

Cormier, Zoe. "No matter what flame retardant is used, it shows up in the environment." *Globe and Mail,* Canada, March 13, 2009.

Coulson, Eric. "New Army Uniform Doesn't Measure Up." Military. com, April 5, 2007.

"Duke Pharmacologist Says Animal Studies on DEET's Brain Effects Warrant Further Testing and Caution in Human Use." Duke Medicine News, May 1, 2002, www.DukeHealth.org.

"Ergon Energy Uniforms 'making workers sick.'" *The Australian,* September 8, 2008.

Faulde, MK, Udelhoven, WM, and Robbins, RG. Contact Toxicity and Residual Activity of Different Permethrin-Based Fabric Impregnation Methods for *Aedes aegypti* (Diptera: Culicidae), *Ixodes ricinus* (Acari: Ixodidae), and *Lepisma saacharina* (Thysanura: Lepismatidae). *Journal Med. Entomol.* 2003;40:935–941.

Faulde, MK, and Uedelhoven, WA. New clothing impregnation method for personal protection against ticks and biting insects. *Int Journal Med Microbiol.* May 2006;296:225–9.

Franklin, Deborah. "Insects, Beware of Clothing That Bites Back." *New York Times,* May 23, 2006.

Hughes, MF., and Edwards, BC. In vitro absorption of pyrethroid pesticides in human and rat skin. *Toxicol Appl Pharmacol.* July 2010;246:29–37.

Issam, C. et al. Effects of dermal sub-chronic exposure of pubescent male rats to permethrin (PRMT) on the histological structures of genital tract, testosterone and lipoperoxidation. *Exp Toxicol Pathol.* April 7, 2010 (Epub ahead of print.)

Kay, Jane. "Study says household dust holds dangerous chemicals." *San Francisco Chronicle,* March 23, 2005.

Kimani, EW. et al. Use of insecticide-treated clothes for personal protection against malaria: a community trial. *Malaria Journal.* July 27, 2006;5:63.

Layton, Lyndsey. "Use of potentially harmful chemicals kept secret under law." *Washington Post,* January 4, 2010.

"Permethrin Facts (Reregistration Eligibility Decision (RED) Fact Sheet)." U.S. Environmental Protection Agency, June 2006. http://www.epa.gov/oppsrrd1/REDs/factsheets/permethrin_fs.htm.

"Permethrin Factory-Treated Flame Resistant ACU's." U.S. Army Center for Health Promotion and Preventive Medicine, Entomological Sciences Program, May 2009. http://chppm-www.apgea.army.mil/DoDIRS/.

Perobelli, JE. et al. Decreased sperm motility in rats orally exposed to single or mixed pesticides. *Journal Toxicol Environ Health A.* January 2010;73:991–1002.

"Pesticide Clothing for Adults and Kids Lack Health Warnings." Action Alert from Beyond Pesticides, August 2, 2004.

Riviere, JE. et al. Gulf War related exposure factors influencing topical absorption of 14C-permethrin. *Toxicol Lett.* September 5, 2002;135:61–71.

Rossbach, B. et al. Uptake of permethrin from impregnated clothing. *Toxicol Lett.* January 15, 2010;192:50–5.

Tanner, CM. et al. Occupation and Risk of Parkinsonism: A Multicenter Case-Control Study. *Archives of Neurology.* 2009;66:1106–1113.

Vanden Brook, Tom. "Troops in Iraq to get fire-resistant uniforms." *USA Today,* December 14, 2006.

Yuan, C. et al. Effects of permethrin, cypermethrin and 3-phenoxybenzoic acid on rat sperm motility in vitro evaluated with computer-assisted sperm analysis. *Toxicol In Vitro.* March 2010;24:382–6.

Chapter 5

"Are Leading Brand Laundry Detergents Environmentally Friendly?" The Laundry Alternative, Inc., http://www.laundry-alternative.com.

Ball, Jeffrey. "Six Products, Six Carbon Footprints." *Wall Street Journal,* March 1, 2009.

"California Bans Toxic Dry-Cleaning Chemical." *Associated Press,* January 26, 2007.

Corea, NV. et al. Fragrance allergy: assessing the risk from washed fabrics. *Contact Dermatitis.* July 2006;55:48–53.

"Eco-friendly options for the laundry." *Myrtle Beach Sun News,* March 18, 2006.

Gillham, Christina. "Nine ways to avoid household toxins." *Newsweek,* October 2, 2008.

"Get rid of chemical fabric softeners: Protect your health and the environment." Fall 2007, http://www.environmentalhealth.ca/special/fall07FabricSofteners.html.

Hake, CL, and Stewart, RD. Human Exposure to Tetrachloroethylene: Inhalation and Skin Contact. *Environmental Health Perspectives.* December 1977;21:231–38.

"Hormone-disrupting contaminants were detected in Laundry Wastewater." The Environmental Working Group, http://www.ewg.org/node/21851.

Johansen, JD. et al. Allergens in combination have a synergistic effect on the elicitation response: a study of fragrance-sensitized individuals. *British Journal Dermatology.* August 1998;139:264–70.

MacIntosh, Helen Suh. "Green Alternatives to Traditional Dry Cleaning." http://www.treehugger.com/files/2007/02/ask_treehugger.php., February 15, 2007.

Prioleau, Cassandra. "Assessment of the Potential for Health Concerns Associated with the Utilization of the Dry Cleaning Solvent, Perchloroethylene." Memorandum to Patricia Adair, Textile Technologist, Division of Combustion and Fire Sciences, U.S. Consumer Product Safety Commission, July 6, 2006.

Chapter 6

"Ancient fabrics, high-tech geotextiles." International Year of Natural Fibres 2009, http://www.naturalfibres2009.org/en/fibres/index.html.

Bond, Annie B. "Effective Ways to Remove Laundry Stains." http://www.care2.com/greenliving/remove-laundry-stains-12-tips.html., November 5, 1999.

"Dressing Green." Union of Concerned Scientists, www.ucsusa.org, June 2000.

Fisk, Umbra. "Advice on natural fabrics vs. polyester." Grist Environmental News and Commentary, July 12, 2004.

Kahlenberg, Rebecca R. "Getting Clean and Green: Earth-Friendly Products Are Going Mainstream, One Shelf at a Time." *Washington Post,* September 17, 2003.

"Making Natural Dyes From Plants." http://www.pioneerthinking.com/naturaldyes.html.

"New Approach of Synthetic Fibers Industry." Textile Exchange, http://teonline.com/articles/2009/01/new-approach-of-synthetic-, January 21, 2009.

"Organic clothing information: Organic cotton, wool, silk, and hemp." Organicnaturenews.com.

Priesnitz, Wendy. "Organic Fibers: Dress Yourself and Your Home with a Conscience." *Natural Life Magazine,* http://www.naturalifemagazine.com/0406/organic_fibers.htm.

Vanderlinden, Colleen. "No stiff jeans, bunchy shoulders, or wrinkled pants." GreenPlanet.com, May 25, 2010.

Chapter 7

"An Overview of Textiles Processing and Related Environmental Concerns." Greenpeace Research Laboratories, University of Exeter UK, June 2005.

Benn, TM, and Westerhoff, P. Nanoparticle silver released into water from commercially available sock fabrics. *Environmental Science Technology.* June 1, 2008;42:4133–9.

Bilberg, K. et al. Silver nanoparticles and silver nitrate cause respiratory stress in Eurasian perch *(Perca fluviatilis). Aquatic Toxicology.* January 31, 2010;96:159–65.

Burke, Myles. "Spray-on clothing in a can to be launched." *London Telegraph,* September 16, 2010.

Carlson, C. et al. Unique cellular interaction of silver nanoparticles: size-dependent generation of reactive oxygen species. *Journal Phys Chem B.* October 30, 2008;112:13608–19.

"Consumer Product Safety Commission Not Ready For Nanotech." Project on Emerging Nanotechnologies, Woodrow Wilson Center, August 21, 2008.

Cumberland, SA, and Lead, JR. Particle size distributions of silver nanoparticles at environmentally relevant conditions. *J Chromatogr A.* December 25, 2009;16:9099–105.

Fabrega, J. et al. Silver nanoparticles impact on bacterial growth: effect of pH, concentration, and organic matter. *Environmental Science Technology.* October 1, 2009;43:7285–90.

Geranio, L. et al. The Behavior of Silver Nanotextiles during Washing. *Environmental Science Technology.* September 24, 2009;43:8113–8118.

Greulich, C. et al. Studies on the biocompatibility and the interaction of silver nanoparticles with human mesenchymal stem cells (hMSCs). *Langenbeck's Arch Surgery.* May 2009;394:495–502.

Griffitt, RJ. et al. Effects of particle composition and species on toxicity of metallic nanomaterials in aquatic organisms. *Environmental Toxicology Chemistry.* September 2008;27:1972–8.

Hussain, SM. et al. In vitro toxicity of nanoparticles in BRL 3A rat liver cells. *Toxicol In Vitro.* October 2005;19:975–83.

Jeng, HA, and Swanson, J. Toxicity of metal oxide nanoparticles in mammalian cells. *Journal Environmental Science Health A.* 2006;41:2699–711.

Kulthong, K. et al. Determination of silver nanoparticles release from antibacterial fabrics into artificial sweat. *Particle Fibre Toxicology.* April 2010;7:8.

McDonough, William, and Braungart, Michael. *Cradle to Cradle: Remaking the Way We Make Things.* New York: North Point Press, 2002.

"New Methods and Tools Needed to Measure Exposure to Airborne Nanomaterials." Project on Emerging Nanotechnologies, Woodrow Wilson Center, April 17, 2007.

Oberdorster, G. et al. Nanoparticles and the brain: cause for concern? *Journal Nanoscience Nanotechnology.* August 2009;9:4996–5007.

Rosas-Hernandez, H. et al. Effects of 45-nm silver nanoparticles on coronary endothelial cells and isolated rat aortic rings. *Toxicol Lett.* December 15, 2009;191:305–13.

Schneider, Andrew. "EPA May Give 1st Approval of Nanosilver for Fabrics." AOL.com, August 18, 2010.

Schneider, Andrew. "The Nanotech Gamble: AOL News' Key Findings." AOL.com, March 24, 2010.

Shavandi, Z. et al. In vitro toxicity of silver nanoparticles on murine peritoneal macrophages. *Immunopharmacol Immunotoxicol.* May 27, 2010 (Epub ahead of print.)

"Silver Beware: Antimicrobial Nanoparticles in Soil May Harm Plant Life." *Scientific American,* August 9, 2010.

Tolaymat, TM. et al. An evidence-based environmental perspective of manufactured silver nanoparticles in syntheses and applications: a systematic review and critical appraisal of peer-reviewed scientific papers. *Science Total Environment.* February 1, 2010;408:999–1006.

About the Authors

For more than three decades Dr. Anna Maria Clement and her husband, Dr. Brian Clement, have directed The Hippocrates Health Institute in West Palm Beach, Florida. It has been hailed by *Spa Management* magazine as "the number one wellness spa in the world."

More than 300,000 people from fifty countries have spent time at Hippocrates to either strengthen their health using the clinic's holistic model, or to heal and recover from illnesses and diseases that mainstream medicine failed to treat. As part of its preventive approach to health, Hippocrates educates its guests about the role that synthetic chemicals play in triggering illness and disease.

The many dozens of celebrity clients who have lent their names in support of the Hippocrates program include the actor Paul Newman, comedian Dick Gregory, musician Kenny Loggins, and Mick Fleetwood of Fleetwood Mac.

Dr. Anna Maria Clement and Dr. Brian Clement lecture on health, healing, and longevity before tens of thousands of people around the world each year. Together and on their own, they have authored a dozen books.

BOOK PUBLISHING COMPANY

since 1974—books that educate, inspire, and empower

To find your favorite vegetarian and soyfood products online, visit:
www.healthy-eating.com

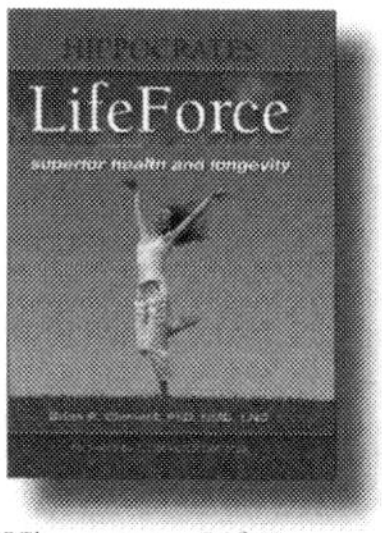

Hippocrates LifeForce
Brian R. Clement, PhD, NMD, LNC

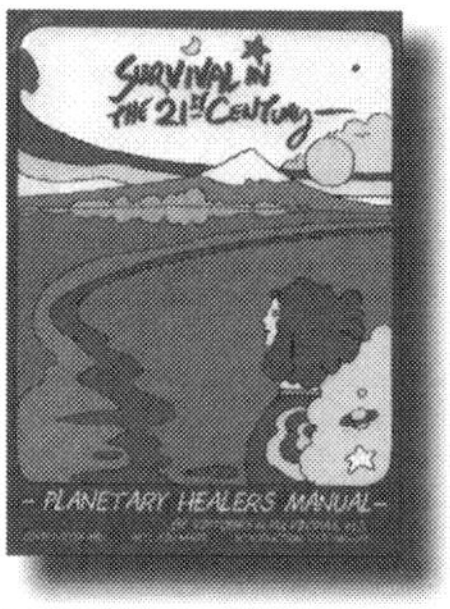

Survival in the 21st Century
Viktoras H. Kulvinskas

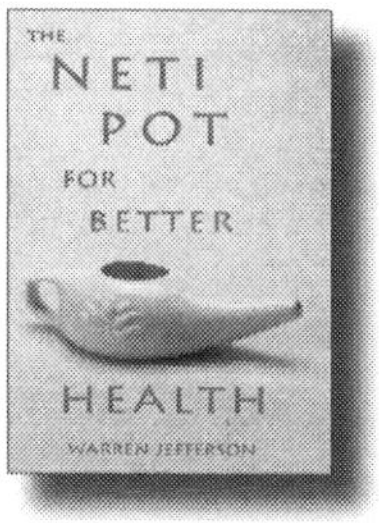

The Neti Pot for Better Health
Warren Jefferson

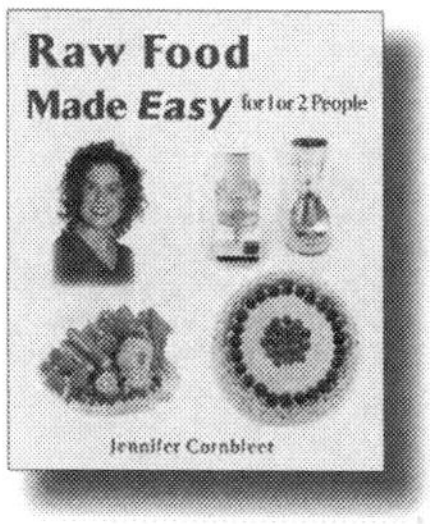

Raw Food Made Easy
Jennifer Cornbleet

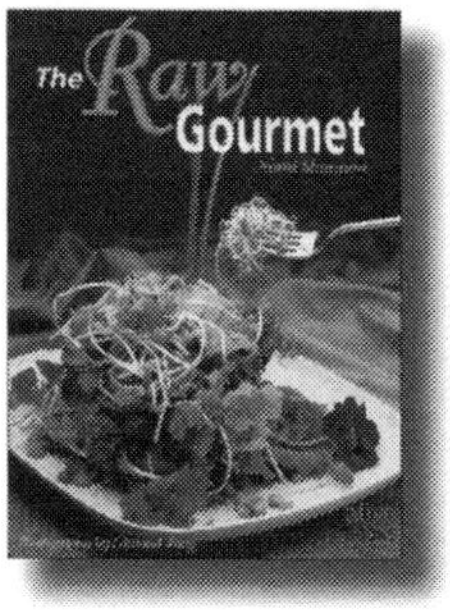

The Raw Gourmet
Nomi Shannon

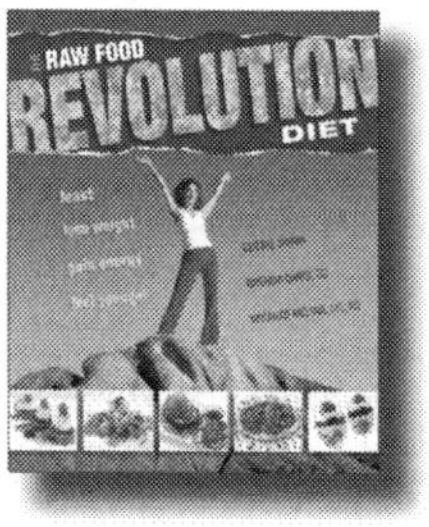

The Raw Food Revolution Diet
Cherie Soria,
Brenda Davis, RD,
Vesanto Melina, MS, RD

Purchase these health titles and cookbooks from your local bookstore or natural food store, or you can buy them directly from:

Book Publishing Company • P.O. Box 99 • Summertown, TN 38483 • 1-800-695-2241

Back Cover Material

The clothes you wear may shorten your life and impact your health.

Did you know that:

- Wearing a bra, especially a tight one, can increase your chance of developing breast cancer.
- Synthetic fibers are such a burn hazard that the U.S. military prohibits troops from wearing them off base.
- Man-made fibers in sportswear can reduce an athlete's competitive edge.
- Close-fitting synthetic underwear can contribute to infertility in men.
- Adequate testing has not been done to determine whether fabric additives, such as insecticides and metals, can safely be in constant contact with human skin.

Man-made clothing fibers, such as nylon, spandex, and Teflon, have only replaced cotton, wool, and silk over the last sixty years. During this time there's been a significant increase in health problems that may be associated with wearing synthetic garments: fertility problems, respiratory disease, contact dermatitis, and cancer.

Killer Clothes reveals the many ways that synthetic clothing, chemicals added to garments, and tight clothing and tight shoes create dangerous problems for human health. Dr. Anna Maria Clement and her husband Dr. Brian Clement, codirectors of The Hippocrates Health Institute, document the rise in health problems that has paralleled the increased use of synthetic clothing fibers. They intend to create wider awareness of the many medical studies—which the media has mostly ignored—showing the harmful consequences to health of wearing synthetic clothing.

Learn:

- what fabrics and chemicals to watch for when selecting clothing
- how to identify deceptive synthetic fabrics
- why to avoid any garment that is advertised as being antishrink, antibacterial, antimicrobial, antistatic, antiodor, antiflame, antiwrinkle, or antistain
- the advantages for chosing natural fabrics
- tips for ecological and health-friendly cleaning

A

B

D

E

F

N

Q

R

S

Books For ALL Kinds of Readers

At ReadHowYouWant we understand that one size does not fit all types of readers. Our innovative, patent pending technology allows us to design new formats to make reading easier and more enjoyable for you. This helps improve your speed of reading and your comprehension. Our EasyRead printed books have been optimized to improve word recognition, ease eye tracking by adjusting word and line spacing as well as minimizing hyphenation. Our EasyRead SuperLarge editions have been developed to make reading easier and more accessible for vision-impaired readers. We offer Braille and DAISY formats of our books and all popular E-Book formats.

Printed in Dunstable, United Kingdom

91336853R00141